Synaptic modification,
Neuron selectivity, and
Nervous system organization

Synaptic Modification, Neuron Selectivity, and Nervous System Organization

Edited By

William B. Levy

James A. Anderson

Stephen Lehmkuhle

LEA LAWRENCE ERLBAUM ASSOCIATES, PUBLISHERS

1985   Hillsdale, New Jersey   London

Copyright © 1985 by Lawrence Erlbaum Associates, Inc.
All rights reserved. No part of this book may be reproduced in
any form, by photostat, microform, retrieval system, or any other
means, without the prior written permission of the publisher.

Lawrence Erlbaum Associates, Inc., Publishers
365 Broadway
Hillsdale, New Jersey 07642

Library of Congress Cataloging in Publication Data
Main entry under title:

Synaptic modification, neuron selectivity, and nervous
  system organization.

  Bibliography: p.
  Includes indexes.
  1. Synapses. 2. Neural transmission. 3. Neurons.
4. Visual cortex. 5. Nervous system. I. Levy,
William B. II. Anderson, James A. III. Lehmkuhle,
Stephen W., 1951–   .
QP364.S97 1985   591.1'88   85-1612
ISBN 0-89859-344-1

Printed in the United States of America
10 9 8 7 6 5 4 3 2 1

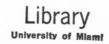

Contents

Contributors

James A. Anderson, Brown University, Department of Psychology and Center for Neural Sciences, Providence, RI 02912

Andrew G. Barto, University of Massachusetts, Department of Computer and Information Science, Amherst, MA 01003

Jean-Pierre Changeux, Neurobiologie Moléculaire et Laboratoire associé au Centre National de la Recherche Scientifique Interaction Moléculaires et Cellulaires, Institut Pasteur, 25 rue du Docteur Roux, 75015, Paris, France

J. D. Cowan, University of Chicago, Department of Biophysics and Theoretical Biology, Chicago, IL 60637

L. N. Cooper, Brown University, Department of Physics, Providence, RI 02912

Nancy L. Desmond, University of Virginia School of Medicine, Department of Neurological Surgery, Charlottesville, VA 22908

Teuvo Kohonen, Helsinki University of Technology, Department of Technical Physics, SF-02150, Espoo 15, Finland

Pekka Lehtio, Helsinki University of Technology, Department of Technical Physics, SF-02150, Espoo 15, Finland

William B. Levy, University of Virginia School of Medicine, Department of Neurosurgery, Charlottesville, VA 22908

P. Munro, Brown University, Department of Physics, Providence, RI 02912

Erkki Oja, Helsinki University of Technology, Department of Technical Physics, SF-02150, Espoo 15, Finland

J. D. Pettigrew, National Vision Research Institute of Australia, 386 Cardigan Street, Carlton, Vic., Australia

C. Scofield, Brown University, Department of Physics, Providence, RI 02912

W. Singer, Max Planck Institute for Psychiatry, Kraepelinstr. 2, 8000 Munchen 40, Federal Republic of Germany

Richard S. Sutton, University of Massachusetts, Department of Computer and Information Science, Amherst, MA 01003

Introductory Remarks

L. N. Cooper
Center for Neurosciences and Physics Department

I want to welcome you to the last in our series of workshops under a Sloan Foundation grant to the Centers for Neural Science and Cognitive Science here at Brown. I'd like to greet everybody and thank you all for coming — some of you from very far away — to be with us in this workshop. I feel somewhat like the host in a Gothic novel who has invited a large number of guests for a weekend. None of the guests has a clear idea of why he was invited until the host begins to tell his stories and says, "One of you will die."

I trust nothing that drastic will happen, but I think it's interesting that the question arises. This is clearly not a workshop organized around a single technique or around a particular piece of anatomy. Rather, it is organized around an idea, or an attempted idea; this idea of course is how modification in single neurons, the behavior of single neurons, can be related to what is known experimentally and can eventually be used as the basis of higher nervous system organization.

To say that one is going to go from the molecular biology of a single synapse to cognitive behavior may seem premature or even absurd — to quote Eric Kandel in an article he wrote some years ago concerning the single synapse and psychotherapy. Frankly, I don't think it's either premature or absurd. As you will see from the progression of the talks, the theme that we're trying to develop begins with the work of Kandel and Castellucci, which indicates that modification at single synaptic junctions in a very simple animal is related to certain behavioral changes. The work of Levy is another and somewhat newer approach that gives very interesting evidence of synaptic modification and is closely related to the work in visual cortex that we'll hear about this afternoon. Although there's not complete agreement among all experimentalists, I think many people would agree that the work in visual cortex clearly shows that input-output relations or the synaptic junctions of individual cells are being modified, the extent of the modification depending on the experience of the animal in its early upbringing. I discussed this matter once with David Hubel, who is not entirely sympathetic to this point of view. He said, "Well, even if you do observe changes, even if you do have plasticity in visual cortex, the main architecture of visual cortex is laid down by genetics." Now that may or may not be the case; I'm not willing to offer a definitive opinion on that. Nonetheless, I do believe that the main interest of the people doing work in the deprivation experiments is not really visual cortex. What it really is is an attempt to see if a kind of plasticity that exists throughout the central nervous system is making itself evident in visual cortex. Even if there are only three cells of visual cortex that show this plasticity, that is an immensely important fact in our attempt to understand the central nervous system. Of course, one can always say that the plasticity in visual cortex is completely different from plasticity elsewhere. That's a possibility. However, it does seem unlikely that nature is so perverse. That has not proven to be the case before, and the reasonable initial working hypothesis is for some kind of simplicity.

The session tomorrow morning will present various theoretical ideas concerning distributive memories and cortical models. In addition, it will include a discussion of how a central set of assumptions can explain much of what is now known about deprivation and normal development of visual cortex and can perhaps also serve as the basis for a theory of higher nervous system organization. In the afternoon we will hear about the Changeux model of how a synapse can modify itself. Following that will be a talk concerning what might be called the difference between local and global controls of modification. On the final morning, we will have a variety of talks on how modification of a single neuron can eventually be related to higher nervous system properties, eventually cognition.

Now that's an immense span, and it's obvious that there are great gaps. However, it seems clear to me that modification must be taking place somewhere in the nervous system and that this modification must have something to do with our experience, or else our memory would really have nothing to do with our past. And it doesn't seem unreasonable — at least it's not without precedent, biologically — that once mechanisms are established, these mechanisms tend to be used over and over again in a variety of different ways. Hence it doesn't seem unreasonable to look for dominating themes and ideas.

In setting up this workshop, we intentionally scheduled relatively few talks. The idea was to try to focus on the theme. In our luncheon discussions, we hope to generate an interaction so that what is said in the talks can serve as a basis for launching a discussion, for arriving at some agreement, some understanding that is different from what we had when we arrived.

I'd like to say a few words, as a theoretician, about how I see the role of theory. First of all, perhaps it's not wrong to compare the central nervous system to something like a Boeing 747. You see, if you had a 747 and you didn't know what it was about — if you'd just come from another planet — it would present an incredible problem to you. You would not know what it was for, what it did, why the seats were there. There are a variety of ways you could go about finding out. You could construct a black box and ask the black box questions to see if this is the sort of thing that the 747 does. You could try analyzing the individual systems. This is not to say that any one approach would necessarily be the final one. But I think that the central idea is that the way one understands a complex system of this kind is to try to see if one can arrive at the underlying principles by which it functions — what it's there for, what it's doing. One tries to trace the evolution of the individual systems because, after all, in the 747, many of the systems really came from the earliest planes; they're just there, fully developed. Perhaps it's not too different in the central nervous system. Many of the elements have come about through evolution, and they somehow interact with each other. At least, the overall principle seems to be that the thing should function and survive. One of the problems that a theorist has in trying to develop concepts is the fact that initial theories almost inevitably seem too simple. With a vast, complicated structure like a 747, any initial theory you have about it seems inadequate because you're not describing all the wires, all the seats, and so on. But it's extremely important to have the deeper understanding that the thing is meant to fly and that the seats are meant to hold passengers. If you can understand *that,* if you can understand that the kerosene is meant as fuel, then the rest of it becomes simple.

I would like to close by saying a word as to how this understanding sometimes comes about. It is often said that what Galileo gave us was the experimental method and that Aristotle and all those foolish Greeks didn't do experiments. Aristotle said that heavy bodies fall faster than light ones. Galileo did experiments and he said, "No, heavy bodies and light bodies fall at the same rate." But Galileo's statement is not only a misconception, it's absolutely false: Anyone who has ever bothered to look knows that heavy bodies fall faster than light ones. Now you may say, "Well, that's air resistance." But think about it for a moment. Aristotle was in fact closer to experience than Galileo. Aristotle very clearly was thinking of objects falling through the air; he knew that resistance retards them so that the heavier falls faster than the lighter. What Galileo did in effect was to move back from experience. What he said was, not that these bodies float for the same length of time, but that the problem is dramatically simplified if we envisage a situation in which all bodies fall at the same rate. He said, "I claim this will be the case at the surface of the earth in the absence of air resistance." Notice how this approach clarifies the question conceptually. It is immensely fruitful to look at things this way.

When I was in college, I took a series of mathematics courses from a member of the Bourbaki School. You have to take mathematics courses from a member of the Bourbaki School to know what that means—no motivation, just one equation after the other. The instructor was a man named Chabrolet. At one point, with an incredible array of formulas on the board, a student dared to ask, "What is that? Professor, what is that line?" Chabrolet answered, "That's a definition." The student said, "Oh, just a definition." And, for the first time that year, Chabrolet paused and said, "Ah, *just* a definition."

In some sense, in mathematics a definition is the whole thing. You may decide you're going to talk about analytic functions, that that's the fruitful way to look at things, but it's inevitable that people will say, "Well, why that rather than something else? That's too simple." Their objections may be correct: One takes a tremendous risk when one does such a thing. But if it works, the gain is a great clarity in which things come together and in which everyone, even those who seem to be working on very different things, can ask similar questions. It seems to me that this is really the way in which scientific progress has been made. Of course it's too much to expect that all of that will occur in these few days: With all the prima donnas that we have here, it's extremely unlikely that we're going to sing in the same key. However, if we manage during the course of these days, even for a moment, to sing the same song, I think we'll have achieved something.

1 Associative Changes at the Synapse: LTP in the Hippocampus

William B. Levy
University of Virginia School of Medicine

One of our primary research goals is to define the rules governing the alteration of synapses. This chapter focuses on our studies of long-term potentiation (LTP) and synaptic modification following convergent, temporally associated neural activity.

The phenomena of LTP were first hinted at by Lømo in abstract form (Lømo, 1966) and were subsequently reported in detail by Bliss and Lømo (1973) and Bliss and Gardner-Medwin (1973). These studies report that delivering brief, high-frequency conditioning pulses to a monosynaptic system results in a long-lasting increase of the synaptic excitation by these afferents upon their postsynaptic cells. Bliss and Lømo argue, as do McNaughton, Douglas, and Goddard (1978) and ourselves (Levy & Steward, 1979), for the synaptic nature of the changes involved in long-term potentiation. McNaughton et al. (1978) and ourselves (1979) argue that LTP is a cooperative phenomenon involving coexcitation of neuronal inputs and outputs similar to a proposal by Hebb (1949). Furthermore, we also argue that, in tandem with this associative rule for potentiation, these same synapses are also governed by a rather specific rule for removing this potentiation (the so-called phenomenon of "depotentiation").

Though in agreement with the research that preceded ours (cited above), this chapter draws mainly from our own data to argue for the synaptic nature of LTP. Further, it defines more precisely the rules governing associative synaptic modifications with the hope that eventually these rules may take a precise mathematical form. Before discussing this topic certain technical aspects of the system are presented, in particular the anatomical and electrophysiological characteristics of the entorhinal projection to the dentate gyrus. LTP in this system is then described in detail in order to adduce the synaptic nature of LTP as an associative form of synaptic modification.

Introduction to the EC–DG System

The studies reported here use the monosynaptic projection from the Layer II cells of the entorhinal cortex (EC) to the granule cells of the dentate gyrus (DG) of the hippocampus. The axons of the Layer II cells project through the lower levels of EC to enter the angular bundle. Via this fiber tract and the perforant pathway, the EC afferents travel over and through the hippocampus proper in order to reach their synaptic targets (i.e., granule cell dendrites) in the molecular layer of the dentate gyrus. In addition to this very large ipsilateral projection, a small, very sparse Layer II EC projection forms synapses in the contralateral molecular layer. The EC afferents are topographically related to the molecular layer of the DG in the sense that the most laterally placed Layer II cells project to the most distal aspects of the molecular layer, whereas cells located in progressively more medial positions across the EC project to progressively more proximal locations in the molecular layer.

Consistent with the monosynaptic nature of this system, a strong afferent volley initiated in the angular bundle (and maximized for the medial EC afferents) results in an ipsilateral DG response with latencies as short as 1.8 msec. (LTP is detected even at these shortest latencies following the proper conditioning paradigm; Levy, unpublished observations.)

In the experiments that follow, the responses are all measured extracellularly and are of two types, the population EPSP (pEPSP) and the population spike. Lømo has shown (1971) with intracellular recording that the monosynaptic response from the entorhinal cortex to the dentate gyrus is depolarizing and excitatory in that it fires the granule cells of the dentate gyrus. Further, these intracellular events of synaptic depolarization and cell firing are well correlated with the responses of the extracellular electrical field. After a powerful discrete stimulation of EC afferents, measurements from the region of active EC–DG synapses register an initial negative voltage (correlated with local excitatory synaptic activation), quickly interrupted by a brief, positive-going wave form (correlated with the active discharge of granule cell somata and axons). As the electrode is advanced from these dendritic regions into the granule cell layer the polarity of these two wave forms reverses. In the region of the granule cell somata, individual action potentials are detected that are in general temporal correspondence to the population spike (pop. spike) response. LTP of the pEPSP slope is equivalently quantified using either the positive- or the negative-going form of the pEPSP (Wilson, Levy, & Steward, 1981). Thus, the extracellular technique can measure both synaptic responses and cell firing.

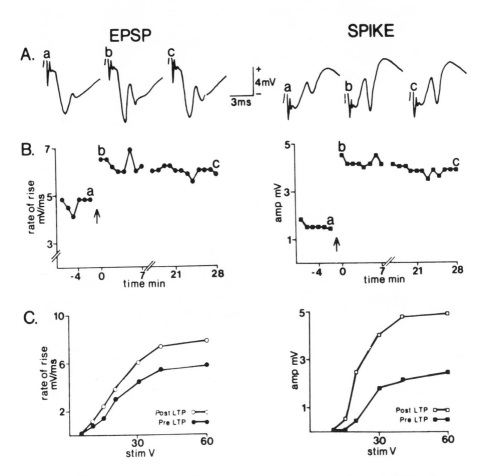

FIG. 1.1 Long-term potentiation (LTP) in the normal ipsilateral temporodentate circuit. The population EPSP (left column) and population spike (right column) were simultaneously recorded. Each response and data point represents a computer average of four evoked potentials. A: sample averaged evoked potentials obtained immediately prior to (a), immediately following (b), and 28 min following (c) 400 Hz conditioning. The responses correspond to points a, b, and c respectively in B.B:LTP of test responses. The test stimulus was delivered at 30 V at a rate of 0.05 Hz. LTP was induced by replacing eight test pulses with 60-V, 20-msec, 400-Hz trains (↑). The break between post-LTP points b and c represents an 8-min period during which the post-LTP input–output function of C was recorded. C: pre-LTP and post-LTP stimulus intensity–response magnitude relationships (input–output functions). (Reprinted from Wilson et al., 1979).

LTP

When high frequency trains are used to activate the EC afferents, there can be a long-lasting increase of the pEPSP and pop. spike subsequently evoked from these conditioned afferents. Figure 1.1 is an example of this LTP. After establishing a baseline to the test pulse (delivered 1/30 sec) a total of 64 pulses are delivered at 8, 400 Hz, 8 pulse trains (one train every 10 sec). Thirty seconds after these conditioning trains, testing is resumed at 1/30 sec. Following the response in time (Fig. 1.1B) reveals a maintained increase of both the pEPSP and the pop. spike. For a group of eight animals, Wilson et al. (1979) showed little difference in the measured LTP at 5 to 10 minutes and 15 to 20 minutes postconditioning. For healthy animals with stable, low noise background activity, my general impression is that if an animal shows

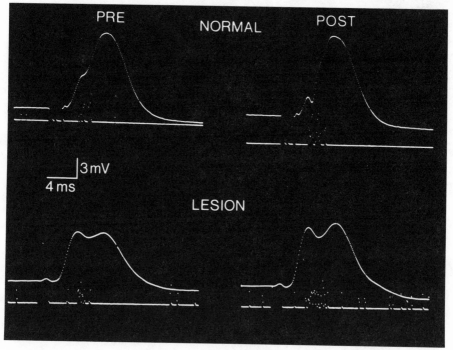

FIG. 1.2   Temporal correspondence of the population spike with cell firing before and during LTP. Pre- and postconditioning responses from one normal (ipsilateral EC–DG system) and one unilateral EC lesioned and sprouted animal (proliferated contralateral EC–DG system) are illustrated. Each trace is the sum of 16 individual responses. Poststimulus time histograms of evoked cell firing (lower trace in each record) were generated by filtering (2–6 KHz bandpass), amplifying, and discriminating responses recorded from the granule cell layer (upper trace in each record). (Reprinted from Wilson, 1981b).

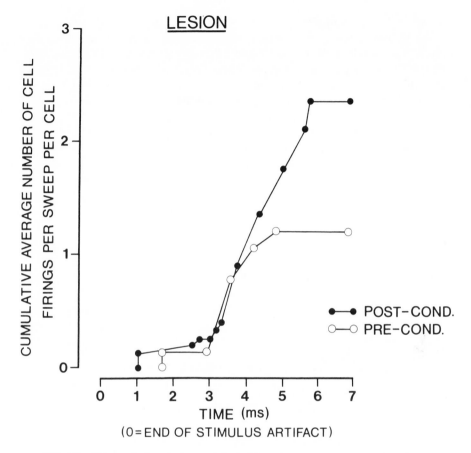

FIG. 1.3   This graph plots the integrated cell firing of the two histograms in the bottom of Fig. 1.2. When plotted in this fashion, it is quite evident that a substantial increase in cell firing has occurred as predicted by the increased population spike seen in Fig. 1.2.

potentiation at 5 minutes postconditioning there is a 95% likelihood that an increase will be present at 10 minutes, and if present at 10 minutes, there is a 95% likelihood that it will be present at 20 minutes, and so on. In several animals we have followed potentiation for as long as 12 hours before terminating the experiment. Other investigators have followed LTP for a day or more (Bliss & Gardner-Medwin, 1973). Thus, very long-lasting increases in synaptic efficacy can result from brief high-frequency conditioning trains.

It is hypothetically possible that an increase of extracellular current flow such as observed with LTP might result from hyperpolarization of the postsynaptic cell's resting potential rather than increased excitatory synaptic activation. However, any such postulated hyperpolarization would cause decreased cell firing and a delay of the pop. spike latency for equivalent pEPSP before and after conditioning. Such results are not the case. Figures 1.2 and 1.3 show that the increased population spike does correctly indicate increased cell firing. Figure 1.4 shows that instead of being shifted to the right, as predicted by the hyperpolarization hypothesis, the input–output curve relating each pEPSP size to its associated pop. spike size is actually shifted to the left. This shift indicates, if anything, that the granule cells are relatively less inhibited after conditioning (cf. Wilson et al., 1981, for a more complete discussion of this shift to the left). Finally, examination of pop. spike latency for equivalent pEPSPs before and after potentiation reveals no delay of this latency (Fig. 1.5). Therefore, none of the evidence is consistent with the hyperpolarization hypothesis. It is concluded that LTP is characterized by larger synaptic excitation, which causes more cell firing (additional evidence for the synaptic nature of LTP is found in the following section).

Associative Synaptic Activation and LTP

The work of McNaughton et al. (1978) begins the systematic investigation of conditioning stimulus intensity upon LTP. These researchers showed that high-frequency conditioning trains to the angular bundle did not evoke LTP unless the intensity surpassed an apparent minimum or critical intensity. In

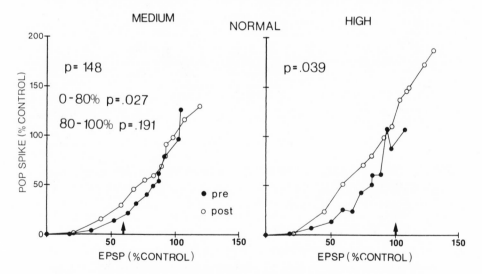

FIG. 1.4 Conditioning-induced changes in population spike/population EPSP relationships. Each group mean population spike is plotted as a function of the population EPSP that generated it. Preconditioning and 5-min postconditioning profiles are illustrated for both medium intensity (left side) and high intensity (right side) conditioning. An arrow (↑) indicates the average population EPSP size evoked at the conditioning stimulus intensity in each plot. (Reprinted from Wilson, 1981b).

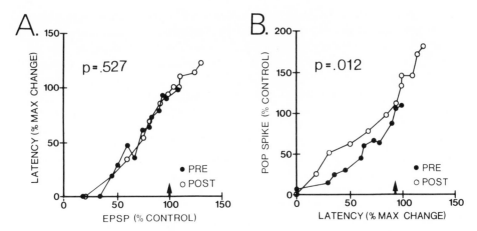

FIG. 1.5   Conditioning-induced changes in the relationship of the population spike and population EPSP to spike onset latency in normal animals. Onset latency was normalized in each animal as the percentage of the preconditioning range from longest (0%) to shortest (100%) latency. In A, the decrease in group mean population spike onset latency is plotted as a function of the population EPSP measure prior to and following high intensity conditioning. In B, population spike size is plotted as a function of the change in onset latency for the same train. An arrow (↑) indicates the size of the population EPSP (A) or the decrease in onset latency (B) at the average conditioning intensity. (Reprinted from Wilson, 1981b).

this type of experiment, a single intensity test pulse is used while conditioning pulse intensity is varied. The implication of this work is of preeminent importance – there is an apparent critical minimum number of coactive afferents required to induce LTP.

In our laboratory Wilson has investigated this phenomenon in some detail. Based on comparisons from eight animals, he found LTP in only two animals when the stimulus intensity was adjusted below that giving a population spike. Increasing the conditioning intensity so that a small pop. spike was obtained resulted in potentiation for six of the eight animals. Finally, using a very powerful stimulus intensity that evoked a large population spike, he was able to demonstrate potentiation in seven of the eight animals (Wilson, 1981).

Generally, this intensity effect is such a simple test that it should always be the initial probe for associatively modifiable synapses. For example we found (unpublished observations) that LTP in hippocampal field CA 1, for both the EC and Schaffer afferents, depends on the conditioning stimulus intensity.

Of relevance to the arguments being presented, at least in our own historical context, is the effect of high-frequency, high intensity conditioning on the synapses of the contralateral EC–DG afferents. These afferents are very sparse in the albino rat (Steward, Cotman & Lynch, 1976) and produce only weak pEPSPs in the DG with little or no pop. spike. For these afferents LTP was not demonstrable in the normal animal. However, with synaptic proliferation of the contralateral EC–DG afferents, via denervation of the relevant DG (the so-called sprouting or reactive synaptogenesis), the contralateral system does show LTP (Wilson et al., 1979).

Available evidence indicates that the sprouted afferents arise via short distance expansion of the terminal field of the normal contralateral system (Steward, 1980). Aside from being significantly more potent (both in terms of pEPSP and pop. spike), the sprouted system has all the other electrophysiological characteristics of the normal sparse contralateral input (cf. Wilson et al., 1979). Thus, until the intensity dependence of LTP became known, it was a bit of a mystery why the sprouted contralateral afferents showed LTP, whereas the normal, contralateral afferents would not. With the existence of intensity-dependent LTP, it was no longer necessary to posit that the sprouted system was functionally different from the normal system, merely that the increase in the number of synapses per parent cell permitted the formation of LTP via enhanced synaptic activity during conditioning. (Table 1.1 shows that LTP is a regular phenomenon of the ipsilateral EC–DG projection and of the sprouted, contralateral EC–DG system but not of the normal contralateral system.)

Actually, there now exist three observations that suggest a minimum coactivity requirement for production of LTP. These three observations are interrelated by the fact that the conditioning stimulus that produces LTP gives a more potent synaptic excitation than the control conditions that do not pro-

TABLE 1.1
Summary of LTP DATA

Response	Number of Rats Showing LTP[a]	Mean % of Baseline ±SE[b]
NORMAL IPSILATERAL		
population EPSP	9/9	141 ± 8.2 (143 ± 7.1)
population spike	8/8	350 ± 97
LESION-INDUCED CROSSED		
population EPSP	8/9	114 ± 1.5 (122 ± 2.6)
population spike	1/7	96 ± 18
NORMAL CROSSED		
population EPSP	0/8	99 ± 3.3

[a]Criteria for LTP were as described in *Methods*.

[b]Post-LTP response amplitudes were averaged over 15 minutes immediately following conditioning for each animal and compared to the average baseline response. To obtain mean % of baseline, results were averaged across animals. Results in parentheses were calculated using the maximal rate of rise of the response.

(Reprinted from Wilson et al., 1979).

duce LTP. The first observation is the requirement for a minimum stimulation intensity during conditioning. The second and third observations stem from comparisons to our consistent failure to produce LTP, using a single conditioning electrode, in the normal contralateral system of the albino rat, even at the highest stimulation intensities. In contrast to this result are the two examples of contralateral projections that show LTP: (1) the sprouted system with its bigger synaptic responses as mentioned above, and (2) our recent observations in the hooded rat showing a normal contralateral pathway of twice the synaptic potency (Levy & Steward, unpublished observations) and twice the synaptic density (Steward, unpublished observations) compared to the albino rat.

Further Evidence Localizing LTP

This section discusses two experiments that use the contralateral EC–DG projections to localize LTP further. The conclusions from the first experiment derive from the collateral nature of the contralateral system.

The evidence that the contralateral EC–DG afferents are collateral branches from ipsilaterally projecting parent afferents is anatomical. Using Golgi methods (unpublished observations, Levy & Desmond) and anterograde HRP methods (in the normal animal, unpublished observations; and Steward, 1980), the contralateral projection appears as an extension of the most anterior portion of the ipsilateral projection. Thin fibers are seen to cross the midline, from one DG molecular layer to the other, in the anterior portion of the dorsal hippocampus where the two sides meet in tenuous contact. In animals with a denervation-induced sprouted contralateral projection, there is strong evidence that the contralateral projection is a collateral of the ipsilateral projection. Using retrograde marking techniques, injections into the contralateral DG label the molecular layer of the ipsilateral DG. More importantly, injecting different retrograde markers into each DG results in labeling of individual EC Layer II cells with both markers (Steward & Vinsant, 1978).

Returning to the simple situation in which the EC–DG afferents are conditioned to produce LTP, we recall from Table 1.1 (see middle portion of Fig. 1.6 for a specific example) that LTP appears only in the ipsilateral system and not in the contralateral system that is simultaneously, and unavoidably also conditioned. (In addition to the data of this table from eight animals, this result has now been replicated in more than 50 other experiments.) Thus, high-frequency activation could not have been the sufficient stimulus for LTP, nor could the changes that mediate potentiation be at the stimulation site or anywhere along the main axon. For these statements to be false, there would have to be LTP in the contralateral system. The alterations mediating LTP must then be localized to nerve endings or their postsynaptic targets. The fail-test S₁→R₁

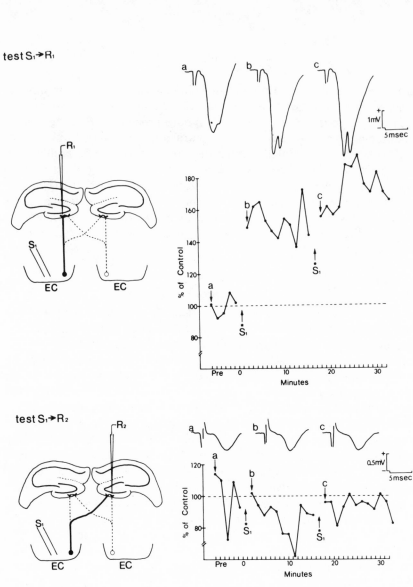

test S₁→R₂

test S₂→R₁

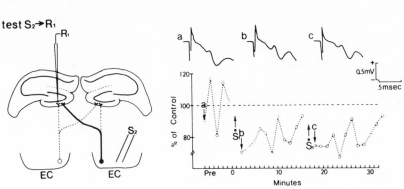

FIG. 1.6

ure to induce potentiation in the collateral system must derive from differential events in one molecular layer versus the other. The obvious difference is the amount of postsynaptic excitation produced by the conditioning stimulation.

The conclusions of the next experiment of this section derive from the convergence between the contralateral afferents on one side and the ipsilateral afferents of the other side in the molecular layer of one DG. The evidence supporting and defining this convergence is: (1) anatomical in the sense that anterograde autoradiography indicates that the synapses of contralateral EC–DG afferents are randomly distributed across the anterior portion of the molecular layer of the DG and must be interspersed among the synapses of the ipsilateral projection, which by itself accounts for over 92% of the total number of synapses of this region (unpublished observation, O. Steward); (2) anatomical and electrophysiological in the sense that the medial to lateral EC-proximal to distal DG topography is maintained by both the ipsilateral and contralateral projections (Levy & Steward, unpublished observations); and (3) electrophysiological in the sense that nonlinear pEPSP summation can be demonstrated between ipsilaterally and contralaterally evoked responses. When found, every cell driven by the contralateral projection is inevitably driven by the ipsilateral projection (see the following sections for other experiments that examine convergence).

Again returning to an experiment in which an ipsilateral projection is conditioned to produce LTP, consider the effect of this conditioning when the convergent contralateral system is tested as is shown in the bottom portion of Fig. 1.6. In such experiments there is no evidence for potentiation of the unconditioned, convergent contralateral system even though the synapses of

---

FIG. 1.6   (*Opposite page*) Effect of ipsilateral entorhinal conditioning stimulation (S_1) on test pulses to the same ipsilateral ($S_1 \rightarrow R_1$) and on both contralateral responses ($S_1 \rightarrow R_2$ and $S_2 \rightarrow R_1$). The top two graphs plot the ipsilateral and contralateral responses, respectively, in response to a test pulse delivered at stimulation site S_1. The bottom graph plots the contralateral response to a test pulse delivered at site S_2. Recording (R_1 and R_2) and stimulating (S_1 and S_2) sites are illustrated in the schematic figure to the left of each graph. For this animal the subscript 1 refers to the left side of the brain, whereas the subscript 2 refers to the right side of the brain. The response being measured is indicated by the darkened pathway in the figure and by the test $S \rightarrow R$ designation and associated traces. An ascendant arrow in the graph indicates the time at which a conditioning series (8, 25 msec trains, one train/10 sec) was given. The location of the conditioning electrode is indicated directly below this arrow. Each descending arrow and associated lowercase letter in the graph indicates the time of the correspondingly labeled response trace. Test pulses of constant intensity are delivered alternately between S_1 and S_2 so that each stimulating electrode is activated once every 20 sec and 10 sec after the other stimulating electrode. Each point is the average of four responses. The control response is determined by the average response value during the time preceding 0 min. For the $S_1 \rightarrow R_1$ response, slope measurements are used. For the $S_1 \rightarrow R_2$ and $S_2 \rightarrow R_1$ responses the initial negative peak was measured. (Reprinted from Levy & Steward, 1979).

this system are no farther than 3 microns from an ipsilateral synapse and are forming synapses on the same postsynaptic cells. Thus LTP must involve a highly specific change. This change, mediating increased synaptic efficacy, cannot be due to generalized chemical changes of the extracellular milieu or changes generalized across the postsynaptic cell (such as resting potential or resting impedance).

Combining the conclusions from both experiments (i.e., the specificity implied by this last experiment and the localization implied by the first experiment) leads to the conclusion that LTP is localized to specific synapses. Those specific synapses would be the ones that were coactive with large amounts of postsynaptic excitation during conditioning. The experiments that follow, showing the associative nature of potentiation, produce further evidence for the specificity on a synapse-by-synapse basis.

Potentiation and Depotentiation of the Normal Contralateral Afferents

Fullest expression of this final conclusion and a more direct example of the associative nature of LTP is shown in experiments using two stimulating electrodes. To give the strongest interpretations to such experiments, the stimulating electrodes should unequivocally stimulate two totally different populations of monosynaptic afferents, one of which is, *by itself*, incapable of being conditioned into a state of LTP. In fact, the ipsilateral afferents of one side and the converging contralateral afferents originating on the other side fulfill the requirements. As already mentioned, conditioning the contralateral afferents alone does not induce potentiation, and conditioning ipsilateral afferents alone does not potentiate the converging contralateral system. However, as predicted by the conclusion of the preceding section, coconditioning of convergent ipsilateral and contralateral projections should result in potentiation of the contralateral system because such conditioning provides presynaptic activity paired with large amounts of convergent synaptic activation.

Figure 1.7 shows the result of such an experiment in which paired conditioning of a strong ipsilateral input with a weak contralateral input produces LTP when the weak input alone is tested. This paired potentiation is consistently observed in spite of the fact that conditioning of the contralateral system alone is ineffective (cf. top portion of Fig. 1.6). Furthermore, this effect is dependent on the intensity of the ipsilateral conditioning stimulus but not on the intensity of contralateral stimulus. So long as an intensity of contralateral stimulation is used that will evoke a measurable response, it is possible to potentiate this response by paired conditioning with the ipsilateral system.

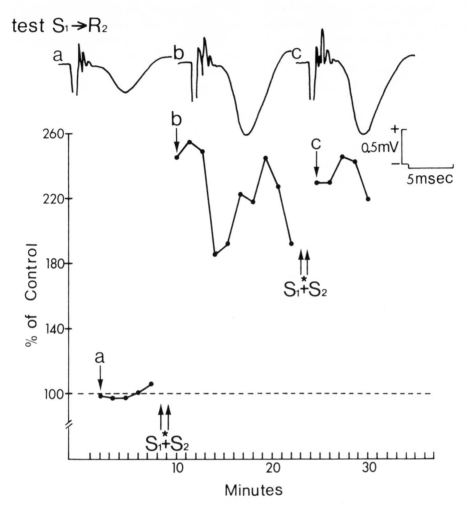

FIG. 1.7 Effect of paired conditioning stimulation $(S_1 + S_2)$ on the contralateral response $(S_1 \rightarrow R_2)$. This is the same animal as Fig. 1.6, and stimulation and recording sites refer to the placements described in Fig. 1.6. The ordinate plots the response to the constant test probe delivered 1/20 sec at S_1. The baseline was established in the time period prior to the combined stimulation and in fact occurred 2 min after the last response of Fig. 1.6. Data are scored as in Fig. 1.6. Notice that whereas neither of the contralateral responses were potentiated by conditioning of S_1 alone (compare effects of $S_1 \rightarrow R_2$ of Fig. 1.6 and $S_2 \rightarrow R_1$ of Fig. 1.6 to Fig. 1.7), paired conditioning trains at $S_1 + S_2$ result in long-term potentiation of the contralateral response evoked by S_1 stimulation. (Reprinted from Levy & Steward, 1979).

Extrapolating from this last result leads to the conclusion that individual synapses can be specifically potentiated if they are coactive with a sufficient amount of convergent postsynaptic activity. Therefore, if the postsynaptic cell is the spatial unit over which convergence is integrated, and because the activity of each cell is a function of the activity of its individual synapses, a large variety of groupings of potentiated synapses has the possibility to form on a cell. Thus, as discussed previously by Anderson (1979), Kohonen (1977), and Cooper, Lieberman, and Oja (1979), a cell-specific and perhaps unsupervised form of concept learning is possible, even from a random network.

In addition to the associative potentiation predicted by Hebb (1949), others (Cooper et al., 1979; Kohonen, 1977; Ranck, 1964; Rosenblatt, 1967; Stent, 1973) predict that there should also be conditions that lead to "depotentiation." Referring back to the bottom two-thirds of Fig. 1.6, it appears that there might be a tendency for nonpairing situations to cause depotentiation, particularly the condition in which the ipsilateral system is conditioned while the convergent contralateral system is unstimulated. Figure 1.8 shows the result of such an experiment upon a potentiated contralateral response (this figure is in fact a continuation of the previous figure). Here it is seen that neither conditioning of the contralateral test system itself nor low intensity conditioning of the convergent ipsilateral system produces depotentiation of the contralateral response. However, when the ipsilateral afferents are conditioned at high intensity (and this happens to be exactly the same intensity used to produce contralateral potentiation via paired conditioning) in the absence of contralateral conditioning, then depotentiation results. Following this depotentiation, potentiation is again induced via the pairing paradigm. In one animal more than 10 cycles of potentiation–depotentiation were demonstrated, although this is not typical. Certainly, though, using the exact paradigm presented here, most animals can be potentiated, depotentiated and, then potentiated again.

In many instances, as in Fig. 1.6, depotentiation is seen prior to experimentally produced potentiation. However, whether or not "depotentiation" can be observed prior to potentiation does not now seem a worthy experimental issue, as the exact state of an animal's synapses at the beginning of an experiment will never be known.

Figure 1.9 summarizes the results of this last series of experiments.

The Monosynaptic Nature of Depotentiation

Since Alger and Teyler's studies of LTP in the sliced, hippocampal explant (1976), there has been little discussion of the possibility of neural loops mediating LTP. We have performed analogous studies of both potentiation and depotentiation to be sure that depotentiation does not depend on neural

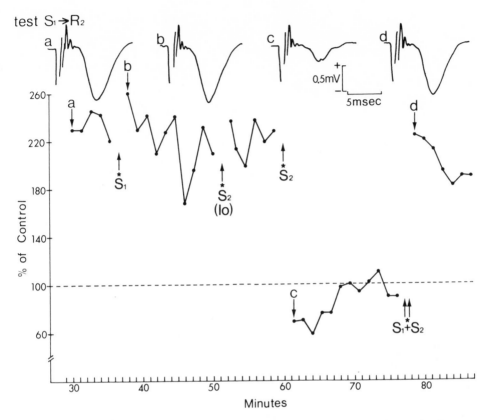

FIG. 1.8   Effect of various stimulation conditions on the potentiated and depotentiated contralateral test response $S_1 \to R_2$. The data are taken from the same animal as shown in the previous two figures and in fact represent a direct continuation of Fig. 1.7. The ordinate plots the response to the same test pulse delivered at S_1 as in Figs. 1.7, 1.8, and 1.6. Nomenclature and electrode placements are as in Fig. 1.6, with the addendum that S_1 (Lo) is a conditioning train using reduced intensity that was subthreshold for a population spike ($S_2 \to R_2$). All other conditioning trains are the same intensity as used previously. (Reprinted from Levy & Steward, 1979).

loops. These studies found both LTP and depotentiation in animals with rather complete knife cuts (Fig. 1.10). These cuts separated the vast majority of Layer II cells from the underlying white matter of the EC thus interrupting the predominant projection path of these cells to the DG.

While on the subject of neural loops it might be added that: (1) there are no reports of axo-axonal synapses in the molecular layer of the DG; (2) in our laboratory, where we have been conducting electron microscopic studies of this region for several years, there is no evidence for such synapses; (3) the rapid onset of pEPSP makes presynaptic inhibition an unlikely mechanism

Associative Potentiation & Depotentiation
(Levy & Steward, 1979)

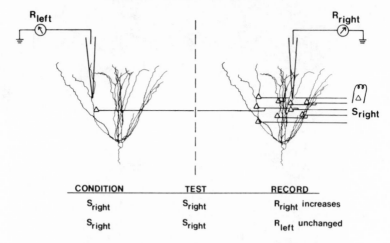

CONDITION	TEST	RECORD
S_{right}	S_{right}	R_{right} increases
S_{right}	S_{right}	R_{left} unchanged

1. Associative potentiation requires coactivity of converging synapses; and even though some synapses potentiate.

2. Collateral synapses without converging activity do not potentiate.

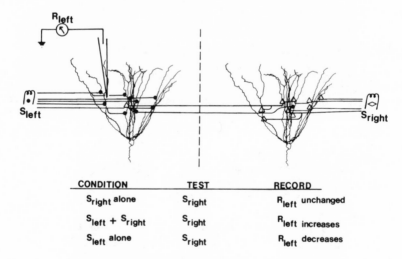

CONDITION	TEST	RECORD
S_{right} alone	S_{right}	R_{left} unchanged
$S_{left} + S_{right}$	S_{right}	R_{left} increases
S_{left} alone	S_{right}	R_{left} decreases

3. An inactive synapse, with neighbors that potentiate, does not potentiate; and if some of these neighbors are convergent.

4. The inactive synapse depotentiates (loses synaptic strength).

CONCLUSION: Modulation of an individual synapse's strength is based upon its activity history relative to the postsynaptic cell's activity history.

FIG. 1.9 Schematic summary of the results of Levy & Steward, 1979.

20

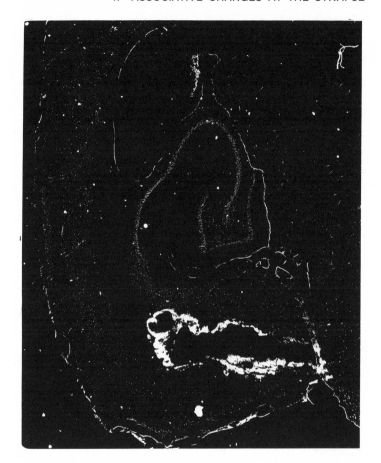

FIG. 1.10   A cresyl violet section showing the results of a knife cut made prior to the conditioning paradigm. This animal had a similar section performed on the other side of the brain and still showed the phenomena of potentiation and depotentiation described by Levy and Steward (1979). At the edge of the knife cut the electrode tract of the angular bundle electrode is visible.

to mediate depotentiation; and (4) the inferred individuality of potentiation/depotentiation as phenomenon modifying responses on a synapse-by-synapse basis would require an inordinately large number of inhibitory presynaptic contacts.

Further Substantiation Using a Partially Sprouted Contralateral Projection

As already seen, convergence arguments are critical to adducing the synaptic specificity of LTP as well as to localizing the site of synaptic integration that is the permissive event for potentiation/depotentiation. In the normal albino rat, demonstration of electrophysiological convergence upon granule cells by the ipsilateral EC–DG input and the contralateral input originating in the opposite EC is sporadic at best, probably because of the small size of this contralateral projection. However, partial EC lesions, and subsequent sprouting, create a system in which two distinctly separate stimulating electrodes can be used to study associative potentiation/depotentiation with convergence regularly demonstrable via several criteria. For these studies one or more of the four types of convergence shown in Fig. 1.11 were demonstrated for each animal studied.

Figure 1.12 shows the average test responses before and after conditioning of the ipsilateral system alone in the partially sprouted preparation. As expected, this conditioning produces depotentiation of the unconditioned contralateral system consistent with the findings already discussed. This improved system with its variety of convergence measures then replicates the results presented in the preceding section.

These same data are also useful for showing that depotentiation of the pEPSP is accompanied by decreased granule cell activation as would be expected if depotentiation represents a true decrease of excitatory synaptic transmission. As shown in Figs. 1.2 and 1.3, the pop. spike of the sprouted contralateral input is associated with and probably represents the envelope of summated granule cell activity. Figure 1.12 shows the decreased pop. spike response accompanying depotentiation of the pEPSP. Therefore we conclude that depotentiation represents decreased excitatory synaptic activity.

Ultrastructural Correlates of Potentiation/Depotentiation

Perhaps the ultimate understanding of these elemental, associative changes will come from ultrastructural and chemical studies describing changes that mediate the altered synaptic efficacies. To this end, we (Desmond & Levy, 1983, Levy & Desmond, in preparation) have just completed a highly quantitative, ultrastructural comparison of the DG for conditioned versus nonconditioned hippocampi. This study finds that in the central region of synaptic activation there are fewer synapses (number per unit volume, the so-called N_V of stereology) with larger active zones. The net total length of postsynaptic densities in this region is unchanged. This result is consistent with the existence of the two opposing processes (i.e., associative potentiation/depotentiation), which are mediated by adjusting the size of the active contact region of each synapse. Associative potentiation would be mediated by the larger synapses, whereas the lost synapses would be the depotentiated population of synapses, which have lost so much active membrane that they are no longer identifiable.

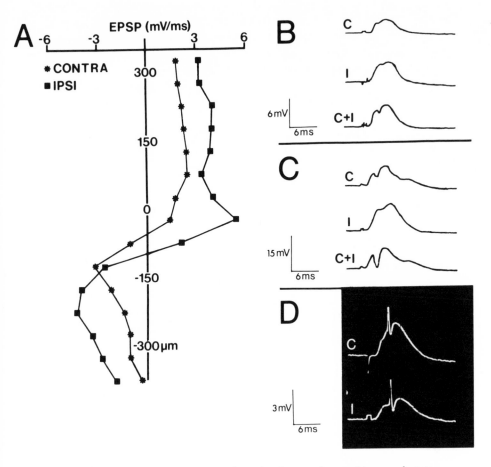

FIG. 1.11 Convergence of surviving ipsilateral and sprouted crossed temporodentate inputs. A. Laminar profile of contralateral (contra) and ipsilateral (ipsi) population EPSP responses recorded in the ventral blade of the dentate gyrus. Ipsi and contra responses were recorded at each side as the electrode was advanced in 50-μm steps through the hilus (positive direction) and the ventral molecular layer (negative direction). Zero (0) indicates the approximate location of the granule cell layer. B. Less-than-linear summation of contralateral (C) and ipsilateral (I) population EPSP responses with simultaneous activation. Responses in B and C are tracings of individual extracellular evoked potentials. C. Greater-than-linear summation of contralateral (C) and ipsilateral (I) population spikes with simultaneous activation. D. Evoked discharge of an isolated granule cell by both contralateral (C) and ipsilateral (I) inputs. Responses are photographs of oscilloscope records. (Reprinted from Wilson et al., 1981).

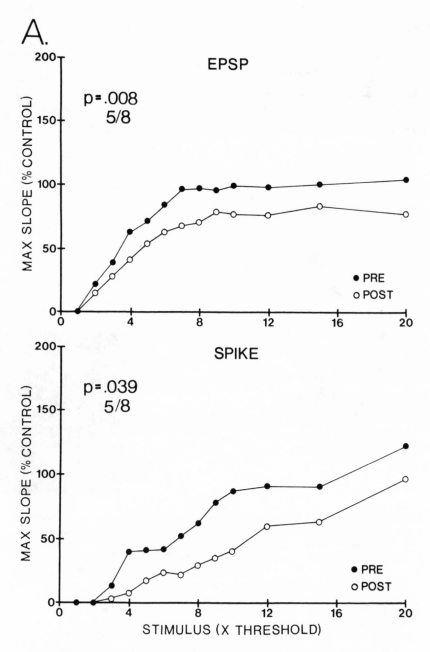

FIG. 1.12 Effects of ipsilateral conditioning on contralateral responses. A. Group mean contralateral response population EPSP and population spike input–output curves recorded prior to (Pre) and following (Post) ipsilateral conditioning. (Reprinted from Wilson et al., 1981).

Further Evidence Supporting Models of Associative Learning Based on Hebbian Rules of Synaptic Modification

A general form of the equations used to describe alteration of synaptic efficacy is

$$\frac{dm_{ij}}{dt} = \epsilon \cdot f(y_j) \cdot g(x_i)$$

where $\dfrac{dm_{ij}}{dt}$ is the change in synaptic efficacy of the synapse formed by the ith afferent upon the jth postsynaptic cell; x_i is the frequency of firing of the ith afferent; y_j is the frequency of the jth postsynaptic cell; $g(\cdot)$ and $f(\cdot)$ are two functions that may or may not yield linear dependencies in x and y; and ϵ is a constant. In this elemental plasticity equation a positive $\dfrac{dm_{ij}}{dt}$ indicates synaptic potentiation whereas a negative $\dfrac{dm_{ij}}{dt}$ means depotentiation.

The following three sections attempt to justify and specify this equation. The section immediately following helps justify the existence of a single equation and postsynaptic excitation as the governing factor of potentiation/depotentiation. Next Hebb's suggestion that postsynaptic cell firing per se (y_j) is the critical variable is called into doubt. In the final section a crude approximation of $g(x_i)$ is made.

Common Events Acting on Postsynaptic Excitation Govern Potentiation and Depotentiation

Experimental motivation for a single plasticity equation to express both potentiation and depotentiation comes from results in which a single manipulation has the same effect on both potentiation and depotentiation. According to the equation such manipulations should effect postsynaptic excitability. Certainly manipulations that control postsynaptic excitation, such as the number of active afferents and their frequency, control the extent of potentiation and depotentiation. Specifically, either low-frequency or low intensity activation of the ipsilateral system is found ineffective for producing potentiation and depotentiation.

Another manipulation that produces a parallel effect on potentiation/depotentiation is commissural stimulation. Buzsàki and Czéh (1981) show that commissural stimulation produces an oligosynaptic inhibition of dentate granule cells. Douglas (1978) reports that properly timed, high-frequency commissural stimulation reduces the production of LTP. We

(Levy & Steward, unpublished observations) have replicated these results and have additionally found that this same commissural stimulation also reduces depotentiation.

Another experiment using commissural stimulation during EC–DG conditioning further supports the notion that $f(y_j)$ represents some form of net postsynaptic excitation. Figure 1.13 shows the effect of commissural stimulation on the pop. spike. Notice that inhibition is greatest shortly after stimulation, but, at long time delays, commissural stimulation actually enhances the EC–DG pop. spike. By using this longer time delay the commissural stimulation, which can block potentiation/depotentiation, turns into a facilitatory influence that lowers the threshold intensity of ipsilateral conditioning stimulation necessary for LTP (Levy & Steward, unpublished observations). These results are consistent with an $f(y_j)$ term that represents the net, summed postsynaptic inhibition and excitation.

The Unit of Integration

We turn now to evidence (Levy & Steward, unpublished observations; see also Douglas, 1978) concerning the neuron as the postsynaptic unit of integration. In general, we have assumed, as did Hebb, that postsynaptic cell firing (y_j) reflects the unit of postsynaptic integration. In fact the results that follow show that other smaller "units" might be considered. In particular, it is possible that individual dendrites or dendritic domains may function as individual associating units. In addressing this possibility, the following paradigm uses a complicated version of the ipsi–contra experiments already described. In this new paradigm there are four stimulating electrodes. Two stimulating electrodes are placed in each EC, one in the medial portion and one in the lateral portion. Using standard mapping methods from recordings taken at various levels of each DG molecular layer, it is first determined that there is a reasonably distant separation (i.e., nonoverlapping voltage maps) between the synapses activated by the medial and lateral electrodes of each side. These experiments can generate four test responses but at this point we need consider only measurements of a single contralateral response.

After establishing a baseline of contralateral test responses, various paired and unpaired conditioning procedures are delivered (conditioning never uses more than two electrodes, testing always uses one stimulating electrode). The question is: Will plasticity-inducing, conditioning stimulation to distal dendritic regions alter the response in proximal dendritic regions? When there is good separation of the responses along the dendrites, independent regions of dendritic processing are found.

Figure 1.14 shows the results of this experiment for the contralateral input to the proximal dendritic regions. Significant response alterations occur only when the spatially convergent ipsilateral afferents are activated. Only the

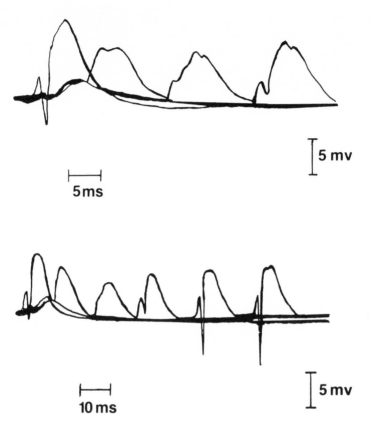

FIG. 1.13 Commissural depression and facilitation of the DG pop. spike to EC stimulation. These recordings were made in the DG granule cell layer so that the negative-going potential breaking up the positive responses presumably represents the envelope of granule cell firing. One stimulating electrode was placed in the angular bundle ipsilateral to the recording electrode. The other stimulating electrode was placed in the contralateral hippocampus between the leaves of the dentate gyrus and was adjusted to maximize the early depression of the pop. spike. Before paired testing, the angular bundle was stimulated at 21 msec delay, evoking the earliest response on the two traces. After the angular bundle stimulation, paired stimulation was delivered at the rate of 1/30 sec. In each pair, the commissural stimulation was delivered at 21 msec delay, and the angular bundle stimulation was delivered with delays ranging from 5 to 70 msec. The top and bottom responses were drawn from a photograph of the traces held by a memory oscilloscope. Notice that between 5 and 30 msec after the commissural stimulation, there is a major depression of the pop. spike. However, around 60 msec after the commissural stimulation, the granule cells are apparently hyperexcitable. In order to show better this late facilitation, the angular bundle stimulation intensity has been reduced slightly in the bottom sequence relative to the top sequence.

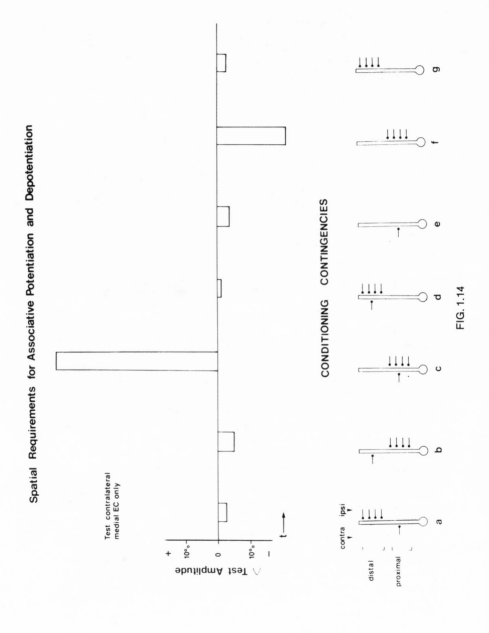

Spatial Requirements for Associative Potentiation and Depotentiation

CONDITIONING CONTINGENCIES

FIG. 1.14

ipsilateral projection to the proximal dendrites is effective for potentiating and depotentiating the spatially convergent contralateral input illustrated in this figure. The ipsilateral projection to the distal dendrites does not control potentiation or depotentiation of the illustrated test response. What is not shown is that this same, apparently, ineffective input is able to potentiate and depotentiate the contralateral input to the distal dendrites whereas the nonspatially converging ipsilateral input is ineffective for this other test system. Therefore, for this experimental situation, the dendritic regions operate in an independent fashion.

Although this study implies that a relatively local unit of postsynaptic integration (i.e., a portion of dendrite) can function as an individual unit of association independent of other portions of the cell, this is not always the case. When large ipsilateral responses of the medial and lateral systems are used for both conditioning and testing, it is quite clear that these two systems can associatively interact across the proximo–distal dendritic axis to produce enhanced LTP (Levy & Steward, unpublished observations; McNaughton, Douglas, & Goddard, 1978). Finally, the dendritic independence observed in the experiment presented here may not be a property of solely the postsynaptic cell but may involve some form of feedforward inhibition. That is, even though such feedforward inhibition is not likely to affect the early stages of the test response, it could easily affect the net postsynaptic excitation during conditioning.

The Time of Integration

Another series of experiments attempted to quantify the coactivity requirement for LTP (Levy & Steward, 1983). The original hypothesis was that the permissive signal for potentiation/depotentiation lasts about as long as there exist substantial amounts of postsynaptic depolarization. Therefore, the ex-

---

FIG. 1.14 (*Opposite page*) Independent processing across the dendritic axis. The bottom portion of this figure indicates the conditioning contingency that immediately precedes each bar graphed above. Four electrodes were used for conditioning stimulation. The two sparse contralateral inputs are indicated by single horizontal lines, whereas the two powerful ipsilateral inputs are each indicated by a group of four horizontal lines drawing up to (i.e., synapsing with) the vertical dendrite of the stick-form granule cell. The relative proximo–distal locations of the conditioned inputs are correspondingly indicated on each stick figure. As usual, conditioning is performed with 8, 8 pulse trains delivered at 400 Hz. Test pulses are then delivered 1/30 seconds for 10 minutes. Each bar represents the difference between the 10-minute average following a particular conditioning contingency and the 10-minute average that precedes it. Thus, a positive value indicates the amount of potentiation a particular contingency induced whereas a negative value is the amount of depotentiation. Notice that only contingencies (c) and (f) effectively alter the test stimulus of the contralateral medial EC. Not shown is the efficacy of conditions (d) and (g) for altering the contralateral lateral EC test stimulus.

pectation was that it would be possible to stagger the "ipsi–contra" paired conditioning protocol, with contralateral conditioning following ipsilateral conditioning by about 10–15 msec, and still observe associative LTP of the contralateral response.

In fact, this hypothesis is the exact opposite of the actual results. Conditioning the ipsilateral afferents prior to the contralateral system consistently results in depotentiation. On the other hand, conditioning the contralateral afferents as much as 20 msec prior (last pulse of contra train to first pulse of ipsi train) to conditioning the ipsilateral afferents results in LTP of the contralateral response. Separating conditioning trains by more than 20 msec rarely resulted in potentiation. The 20-msec interval produced potentiation distinctly inferior to that produced by the nearly simultaneous trains normally used for inducing LTP. Such data argue that the coactivity requirement is not absolute and that an integration period of about 20 msec might exist. Following this line of thought, this result further suggests that individual postsynaptic elements might possess temporal integrating mechanisms (e.g., chemical reactions) that convert synaptic activity into a usable form for only approximately 20 msec. With repetitive synaptic activity more often than once per 20 msec, a form of postsynaptic integration takes place that would be the postsynaptic expression of x_i.

A First-Order Approximation of $g(x_i)$

The simplest form of $g(x_i)$ consistent with the preceding equation and the potentiation/depotentiation characteristics so far described of the EC–DG system is $g(x_i) - (x_i - b)$ where b is some constant. The difference $(x_i - b)$ implies that, given a positive value for $f(y_j)$, potentiation will occur when x_i is greater than b, and depotentiation will occur when x_i is less than b.

Although we have no strong, direct measure of $f(y_j)$, we propose that $f(y_j)$ takes on positive values when a powerful ipsilateral conditioning stimulation is used (i.e., a high-frequency, high intensity conditioning train that is capable of LTP by itself). On the other hand, the conditioning frequency of the contralateral afferents is assumed nearly to approximate x_i while not significantly adding to $f(y_j)$ at any frequency. With these assumptions we can titrate the value of b by pairing ipsilateral stimulation with a variety of contralateral conditioning frequencies. When the contralateral conditioning frequency exceeds b, potentiation results. When the contralateral conditioning frequency is less than b, depotentiation will result.

Using this method, Fig. 1.15 shows that b is greater than 20 Hz but less than 100 Hz. Although not statistically significant, a more adventuresome experiment titrated b as greater than 39 Hz and less than 77 Hz. Such values seem reasonable, considering that the results of the previous section predict a value of b somewhat less than 50 Hz (cf. Levy, Brassel and Moore, 1983, for more details).

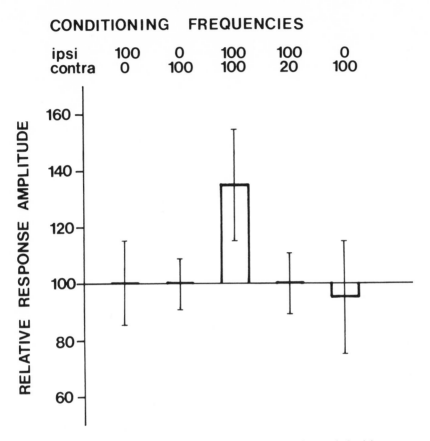

FIG. 1.15   Titration of b. This experiment assumes that the elemental plasticity equation takes the form of $\Delta m = f(y)(x - b)$. $f(y)$ is assumed to be positive because the high intensity ipsilateral stimulus is itself capable of undergoing potentiation. b is assumed to be constant so that when x (the frequency of the contralateral input) is larger than b, potentiation will result, and when x is smaller than b, depotentiation should result. The successive conditioning contingencies are indicated at the top of the figure. All conditioning trains contain 20 pulses regardless of frequency. When paired, ipsi- and contralateral trains always end together. Each bar represents the average contralateral response measured over a period of 12 minutes testing 1/30 seconds. As expected, potentiation of the contralateral response requires coconditioning with the ipsilateral input. On the other hand, using the same number of pulses but slowing down the rate of contralateral stimulation during coconditioning produces depotentiation. These results argue for $20 < b < 100$ Hz.

Finally, we must admit this view of b as a constant is somewhat naive. This is especially emphasized when we consider certain asymptotic predictions of this equation. The predictions that a repeatedly depotentiated excitatory synapse should be converted to an inhibitory synapse (i.e., take on negative values) or, on the other hand, that a repeatedly potentiated synapse should grow in strength without bounds certainly contradict some basic biological intuitions. However, by replacing b with a variable that changes in proportion to m, a satisfactorily bounded form of behavior is obtained. For instance,

$$\frac{dm}{dt} = \epsilon y(ax - m)$$

where a and ϵ are constants, does quite well for our purposes.

In summary then, with the demonstration of synapses that associatively potentiate and depotentiate, it has become possible to begin crude measurements of their quantitative properties. Hopefully, this experimental approach, interacting with relevant mathematical models, will lead to a new dimension of understanding brain functions.

ACKNOWLEDGMENTS

The research reported in this chapter is the result of collaborative efforts with Dr. Oswald Steward, various graduate students including Dr. R. W. Wilson, Mr. Scott Lasher, Mr. Scott Moore, Mr. Paul Munro, and Dr. N. L. Desmond. Supported in part by NIH grants NS12333 to O. Steward and NS15488 to W. B. Levy.

REFERENCES

Alger, B. E., & Teyler, T. J. Long-term and short-term plasticity in the CA1, CA3, and dentate regions of the rat hippocampal slice. *Brain Res.,* 1976, *110,* 463–480.

Anderson, J. A. Parallel computation with simple neural networks. *Cognition & Brain Theory,* 1979, *3,* 45–53.

Bliss, T. V. P., & Gardner-Medwin, A. R. Long-lasting potentiation of synaptic transmission in the dentate area of the unanaesthetized rabbit following stimulation of the perforant path. *J. Physiol.,* 1973, *232,* 357–374.

Bliss, T. V. P., & Lømo, T. Long-lasting potentiation of synaptic transmission in the dentate area of the anaesthetized rabbit following stimulation of the perforant path. *J. Physiol.,* 1973, *232,* 331–356.

Buzsaki, G., & Czeh, G. Commissural and perforant path interactions in the rat hippocampus: Field potentials and unitary activity. *Exp. Brain Res.,* 1981, *43,* 429–438.

Cooper, L. N., Liberman, F., & Oja, E. A theory for the acquisition and loss of neuron specificity in visual cortex. *Biol. Cybernetics,* 1979, *33,* 9–28.

Desmond, N. L., & Levy, W. B. Synaptic correlates of associative potentiation/depression: an ultrastructural study in the hippocampus. *Brain Res.,* 1983, *265,* 21–30.

Douglas, R. M. Heterosynaptic control over synaptic modification in the dentate gyrus. *Soc. for Neurosci.*, 1978, *4*, 470.

Hebb, D. O. *The organization of behavior.* New York: Wiley, 1949.

Kohonen, T. *Associative memory: A system — theoretical approach.* New York: Springer-Verlag, 1977.

Levy, W. B., Brassel, S. E., & Moore, S. D. Partial quantification of the associative synaptic learning rule of the dentate gyrus. *Neuroscience,* 1983, *8*, 799–808.

Levy, W. B., & Steward, O. Synapses as associative memory elements in the hippocampal formation. *Brain Res.,* 1979, *175*, 233–245.

Levy, W. B., & Steward, O. Temporal contiguity requirements for long-term associative potentiation/depression in the hippocampus. *Neuroscience,* 1983, *8*, 791–797.

Lømo, T. Frequency potentiation of the excitatory synaptic activity in the dentate area of the hippocampal formation. *Acta Physiol. Scand.,* 1966, Suppl. 277, 1966–68.

Lømo, T. Patterns of activation in a monosynaptic cortical pathway: The perforant path input to the dentate area of the hippocampal formation. *Exp. Brain Res.,* 1971, *12*, 18–45.

McNaughton, B. L., Douglas, R. M., & Goddard, G. V. Synaptic enhancement in fascia dentata: Cooperativity among coactive afferents. *Brain Res.,* 1978, *157*, 277–293.

Ranck, J. B., Jr. Synaptic "learning" due to electroosmosis: A theory. *Science,* 1964, *144*, 187–189.

Rosenblatt, F. Recent work on theoretical models of biological memory. In J. T. Tou (Ed.), *Computer and information sciences — II.* New York: Academic Press, 1967, 33–56.

Stent, G. S. A physiological mechanism for Hebb's postulate of learning. *Proc. Nat. Acad. Sci., USA,* 1973, *70*, 997–1001.

Steward, O. Trajectory of contralateral entorhinal axons which reinnervate the fascia dentata of the rat following ipsilateral entorhinal lesions. *Brain Res.,* 1980, *183*, 277–289.

Steward, O., Cotman, C., & Lynch, G. A quantitative autoradiographic and electrophysiological study of the reinnervation of the dentate gyrus by the contralateral entorhinal cortex following ipsilateral entorhinal lesions. *Brain Res.,* 1976, *114*, 181–200.

Steward, O., & Vinsant, S. L. Collateral projections of cells in the surviving entorhinal area which reinnervate the dentate gyrus of the rat following unilateral entorhinal lesions. *Brain Res.,* 1978, *149*, 216–222.

Wilson, R. C. Changes in the translation of synaptic excitation to dentate granule cell discharge accompanying long-term potentiation. I. Differences between the normal and reinnervated dentate gyrus. *J. Neurophysiol.,* 1981, *46*, 324–338. (a)

Wilson, R. C. *Functional consequences of the morphological and physiological modification of synapses and circuits in the hippocampal formation of the rat.* Doctoral dissertation, University of Virginia, 1981. (b)

Wilson, R. C., Levy, W. B., & Steward, O. Functional effects of lesion-induced plasticity: Long-term potentiation in normal and lesion-induced temporodentate connections. *Brain Res.,* 1979, *176*, 65–78.

Wilson, R. C., Levy, W. B., & Steward, O. Changes in the translation of synaptic excitation to dentate granule cell discharge accompanying long-term potentiation. II. An evaluation of mechanisms utilizing the dentate gyrus dually innervated by surviving ipsilateral and sprouted crossed temporodentate inputs. *J. Neurophysiol.,* 1981, *46*, 339–355.

2

Hebbian Modification of Synaptic Transmission as a Common Mechanism in Experience-Dependent Maturation of Cortical Functions.

W. Singer
Max-Planck-Institute for Brain Research

Restricting visual experience during early postnatal development leads to profound and permanent alterations of cortical functioning. Depending on the deprivation procedure, cells in the visual cortex may lose their binocular connections and then respond exclusively to either of the two eyes; they may also lose or fail to develop their characteristic selectivity for the orientation and the direction of movement of contours or they may acquire these latter properties in abnormal proportions; and, finally, they may become entirely unresponsive to retinal stimulation. Thus, the characteristic response properties of cortical neurons develop and consolidate only when visual experience is available and not disturbed.

In this chapter I summarize evidence in support of the hypothesis that experience-dependent maturation and modification of cortical functions result from a selection process that augments the specificity of neuronal interactions. Early proliferation of neuronal connections is assumed to provide a redundant, only loosely specified Anlage of excitatory connections, which is then specified further according to functional criteria. This specification is thought to consist of activity-dependent selection, whereby particular subsets of excitatory connections increase their efficiency and consolidate while others weaken and eventually retract from their target. The criteria of selection appear to closely resemble those postulated by Hebb (1949) for adaptive synaptic connections; Hebb assumed that afferents increase their gain and consolidate when the probability is high that they are active in contingency with the postsynaptic cell, whereas their gain decreases when this probability is low (i.e., when the afferent pathways are silent while the postsynaptic cell is activated). In extension of these classical rules, recent data indicate that the experience dependent modifications are in turn gated by additional, probably hierarchically organized, control systems. In order to induce Hebbian modifications, retinal signals must not only match the receptive field properties of the cells in the striate cortex but must in addition be adequate in the more global context of polymodal and visual-motor integration. Moreover, the retinal signals need to be processed by an awake brain and have to be attended to.

Experience–Dependent Modifications at the Level of Binocular Convergence

By the time kittens open their eyes most neurons in the visual cortex respond to stimulation of both eyes, and with normal visual experience this condition is maintained (Hubel & Wiesel, 1962, 1963). However, when signals from the two eyes are incongruent, either because one eye is occluded (Wiesel & Hubel, 1965) or because the images on the two retinae are not in register — as is the case with strabismus (Hubel & Wiesel, 1965), cyclotorsion (Blakemore, Van Sluyters, Peck, & Hein, 1975; Crewther, Crewther, Peck, & Pettigrew, 1980; Yinon, 1975), or anisometropia (Blakemore & Van Sluyters, 1974; Wolfe & Owens, 1979) — cortical cells lose their binocular receptive fields. In the first case they stop responding to the deprived eye; in the other cases they segregate into two approximately equally large groups, one responding exclusively to the ipsilateral and the other exclusively to the contralateral eye. In both cases the loss of binocularity is mainly due to decoupling of thalamocortical afferents from their respective cortical target cells. This follows from two findings: First, in cats, binocular convergence occurs already at the level of cells connected directly to geniculate afferents (Birk & Singer, in preparation). Second, analysis of field potentials indicates that transmission failure actually occurs already at the level of thalamocortical synapses and is due to a real decrease of synaptic inward currents rather than to an increase of interocular inhibition (Mitzdorf & Singer, 1980; Singer, 1977b). During the critical period of early development, these changes are fully reversible indicating, that the efficacy of transmission does not only decrease but can also increase as a function of retinal stimulation (Blakemore & Van Sluyters, 1974; Wiesel & Hubel, 1965). Both impairment and improvement of excitatory transmission appear to depend on responses of the postsynaptic target cells. If the latter fail to respond to signals from either of the two eyes, changes in transmission do not occur even if the pathways from one eye are much more active than those from the other. If, for example, one eye is occluded lighttight while the other is stimulated with flashes of diffuse light, the ocular dominance of cortical cells does not change (Singer, Rauschecker, & Werth, 1977). The most probable reason is that the postsynaptic neurons in striate cortex cannot respond to changes in ambient illumination. Conversely, when one eye is occluded and the other exposed to contours of only a single orientation, differential gain changes occur only at junctions with those postsynaptic cells that are capable of responding to the signals conveyed by the open eye (Rauschecker & Singer, 1979; Singer, 1976). For these cells the efficiency of afferents from the stimulated eye increases, whereas that of afferents from the deprived eye decreases. Cells, by contrast, whose orientation preference does not correspond to the orientations seen by the stimulated eye cannot respond to activity from this eye and do not change their ocular dominance. Here, the afferents from the stimulated eye, even though they are much more active than those from the deprived eye, do not increase their efficiency at the expense of the latter.

The results of these and related experiments (Rauschecker & Singer, 1981) made it possible to formulate three basic rules which have proved sufficient to account for the results of most if not all deprivation experiments published so far. These rules closely resemble those postulated by Hebb (1949) for adaptive neuronal connections and can be summarized in the following way: (1) the gain of a synaptic connection increases whenever the afferent fibre is active in contingency with the postsynaptic target; (2) the gain decreases when the postsynaptic target is active while the presynaptic terminal is silent; and (3) irrespective of the amount of activation of presynaptic terminals, differential gain changes do not occur when the postsynaptic cell is inactive (Fig. 2.1). Whether the required postsynaptic response has to consist of action potentials, or whether the important parameter is the level of dendritic depolarization is still unclear. As discussed later, indirect evidence is actually in support of the latter assumption.

As can easily be seen these activity-dependent changes result in what appears as competition between converging pathways. Whenever afferent pathways convey activity patterns that are out of phase, those connections that have the highest probability of being active in contingency with the postsynaptic cell (Fig. 2.1) will increase their gain and consolidate. Usually this condition is fulfilled for pathways that drive the postsynaptic cell most effectively, either because the activity patterns conveyed by these afferents conform best with the receptive field properties of the postsynaptic cell or because their initial coupling is strongest. In contrast, pathways that have a lower probability of being active in contingency with the postsynaptic cell will decrease their gain and eventually become entirely ineffective. Such is usually the case for pathways that are less effective in driving the postsynaptic cell, either because they are deprived and therefore convey less activity or because their initial coupling with the postsynaptic target cell is

RULES FOR SYNAPTIC MODIFICATION

state of afferent pathway	active	inactive	active or inactive
state of postsynap- tic element	active	active	inactive
change of synaptic gain	increase	decrease	no change

EXAMPLES

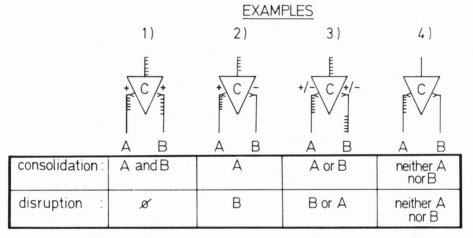

	1)	2)	3)	4)
consolidation :	A and B	A	A or B	neither A nor B
disruption :	∅	B	B or A	neither A nor B

FIG. 2.1 Rules for activity dependent modifications of neuronal connectivity in the developing visual cortex. Example 1: Afferences A and B are active simultaneously and in contingency with postsynaptic target C. Example 2: Only afference A is active in contingency with C, afference B is inactive. Example 3: Both afferences A and B are active but not simultaneously; C is responding to both inputs. Example 4: C is inactive; the state of afferences A and B is irrelevant, changes in gain do not occur.

weaker, or because they convey activity that does not match the receptive field properties of the target cell. There is only one condition in which less efficient afferents are not subject to competition, and this is when they happen to be active in contingency with the more efficient afferents. Profiting from the postsynaptic responses to the dominant input, these afferents may now increase their gain and consolidate as well.

It follows from these considerations that among two converging pathways conveying identical but temporally incongruent activity the pathway with tighter initial coupling will consolidate at the expense of the other. Such a condition is fulfilled in the case of strabismus: the signals conveyed from the two eyes are virtually identical but they are out of phase. In Area 17, initial coupling of afferents converging from the two eyes is approximately symmetrical. Even without visual experience the numbers of cells dominated by the ipsi- or the contralateral eye are about equal (Hubel & Wiesel, 1963; Imbert & Buisseret, 1975). In Area 18, by contrast, there appears to be a natural bias in favour of the respective contralateral eye. From the foregoing prediction we expect that strabismus should lead to very different ocular dominance distributions in the two areas. In both areas cells should become monocular. However, in Area 17 about an equal number of cells should respond to either the contra- or the ipsilateral eye, whereas in Area 18 the vast majority of cells should react to the contralateral eye only. Here, the ocular dominance distribution should be as if the respective ipsilateral eye had been deprived of contour vision altogether. Recent experiments demonstrate that this is in fact the case (Birk & Singer, in preparation, see also Fig. 2.2).

Experience–Dependent Modifications of Orientation Selectivity

In 3-week-old kittens reared without visual experience, a substantial number of striate cortex cells possess a preference for stimulus orientation (Buisseret & Imbert, 1976; Hubel & Wiesel, 1963; Sherk & Stryker, 1976). With increasing duration of visual deprivation, the percentage of these cells decreases, whereas it increases to nearly 100% with normal visual experience (Buisseret & Imbert, 1976). In the latter case, cells with preferences for horizontal, vertical, and oblique orientations are about equally frequent. When, however, the kitten experiences only contours of a single orientation, the majority of cortical cells adopt preferences for this orientation (for a review of the extensive literature see Rauschecker & Singer, 1981). Two recent studies, one based on single-cell recording (Rauschecker & Singer, 1981) and the other on deoxyglucose mapping of orientation columns (Singer, Freeman, & Rauschecker, 1981), converge in the conclusion that also such experience-dependent distortions in the distribution of orientation preferences can be accounted for by Hebbian competition between converging excitatory pathways. The main finding of the deoxyglucose study was that restricting visual experience to a single orientation had only little influence on the development of the orientation column system within Layer IV but produced massive distortions of the columnar system within nongranular layers. Although cells responding to inexperienced orientations were still present within Layer IV and were grouped within regularly spaced bands, activity from these cells was no longer relayed to cells in supra- and infragranular layers. By contrast, activity of Layer IV cells whose orientation preference corresponded to the experienced orientations was now relayed not only to nongranular cells located above and below the active zones in Layer IV but spread tangentially to adjacent cells (Fig. 2.3). Thus, the columns encoding the experienced orientation had expanded into the territory of the deprived columns from which the

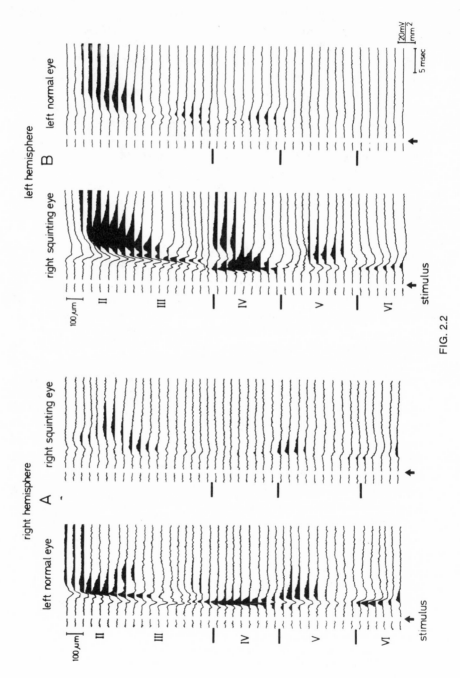

FIG. 2.2

40

latter had withdrawn. In this respect the reorganization of the orientation column system after orientation deprivation closely resembles the reorganization of the ocular dominance columns after monocular deprivation (Hubel, Wiesel, & LeVay, 1977). Only the site of competition appears to be different: In the case of monocular deprivation, competition occurs where afferents from the two eyes converge onto the common cortical target cells, which are located mainly in Layer IV. In the case of orientation deprivation, competition is likely to occur at the level where axons from orientation selective Layer IV cells converge onto second-order target cells that are located mainly in nongranular layers. The spread of activity from the non-deprived Layer IV cells into the territory of the adjacent deprived orientation columns indicates that the intracortical connections between first and second order cells diverge and overlap as is the case for most axonal projections. If these axons compete for the second-order cells according to the rules specified previously, restricting visual experience to a single orientation will lead to an expansion of adequately stimulated columns and to shrinkage of the deprived orientation columns, the latter becoming restricted to the clusters of first-order cells in Layer IV. Conversely, it can easily be seen that normal experience with contours of all orientations will assure that all cells within cylinders orthogonal to the cortical lamination adopt the same orientation preferences as the first order cells contained within these cylinders (Fig. 2.4). The only additional prerequisite for the development of such an orderly arrangement is that, prior to experience, coupling of first order cells onto second order cells is tightest along trajectories perpendicular to the cortical lamination and decreases with tangential distance from these lines. As discussed in detail previously (Singer et al., 1981) both anatomical and physiological data suggest that this is the case. Thus, even prior to experience cells located along lines perpendicular to the cortical lamination can be expected to prefer similar orientations, a conjecture that appears to be in agreement with electrophysiological data (Sherk & Stryker, 1976). However, because of divergence and

---

FIG. 2.2 (*Opposite page*) Current source density distributions measured in area 18 of a strabismic cat after electrical stimulation of the optic nerves. Field potential responses were recorded with a micropipette at 50 μm intervals from white matter up to the pial surface and averaged over 20 stimuli. The current source densities were calculated from field potentials (P n − 4, Pn, Pn + 4) separated by 200 μm, respectively. The depth location of individual current traces is indicated by the scale on the left upper corner and their laminar distribution by the laminar borders on the left margin. The hatched upward deflections of the traces correspond to current sinks and reflect mainly inward current at excitatory synapses; thus, the short latency sinks in layers IV and VI result from monosynaptic activation of cortical target cells by geniculate afferents while the later sinks reflect polysynaptic activity. Comparison of the current source density profiles in the two hemispheres shows that afferences from the respective ipsilateral eye produce much weaker synaptic currents than those from the contralateral eye. This indicates that competitive processes have suppressed the respective ipsilateral connections in both hemispheres.

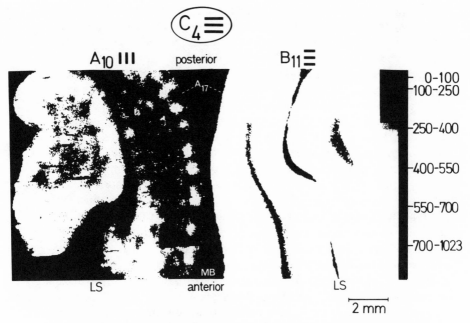

FIG. 2.3   Orientation columns in striate cortex of a kitten (C₄) who had experienced only horizontally oriented contours. To demonstrate the topography of orientation columns the kitten was injected with ¹⁴C-deoxyglucose and then one hemisphere was stimulated with vertical (A 10) and the other with horizontal (B 11) contours. The autoradiographs A 10 and B 11 are from horizontal sections through the occipital pole of the two hemispheres. The plane of the sections is perpendicular to the lamination of area 17. The optical density of the autoradiographs has been quantified with an image processing system (scale on right margin), bright tones corresponding to high optical density. Comparison of the two hemispheres reveals considerably more activity in the hemisphere which, after application of the deoxyglucose pulse, has been stimulated with the same orientation as that experienced previously (B 11). On this side isolated columns are barely distinguishable because they have expanded and are confluent. By contrast, on the other side, zones of increased activity are well segregated from each other and confined essentially to the granular layer of area 17. Thus, cells which are responsive to orientations orthogonal to those which have been experienced previously are still grouped in regularly spaced clusters within layer IV but activity is no longer relayed to more superficial and deeper layers (from Singer et al., 1981).

overlap of connections converging from adjacent first order cells onto second order cells, the orientation tuning of the latter should initially be broad. Only when experience-dependent gain changes have led to selective stabilization of afferents to second-order cells that originate exclusively from first-order cells with identical orientation preference, tuning of second-order cells will become as narrow as that of the prespecified first-order cells. Because of initially tighter coupling the vertically ascending axons possess a competitive advantage and will consolidate preferentially, thus assuring that all cells along lines perpendicular to the cortical lamination adopt or continue to have the same orientation preference as the prespecified first order cells in Layer IV. The functional implications of experience dependent selection of excitatory connections at this level of cortical processing will be discussed at the end of this chapter. For the moment it is sufficient to note that such a selection process allows convergence of numerous first order cells onto a common second order cell without the latter losing its selectivity for stimulus orientation.

Experience–Dependent Modifications of Tangential Interactions

Further indications for modifications of intracortical connections come from experiments in which kittens had selective experience with slowly drifting vertically oriented gratings of constant spatial frequency. In striate cortex of these kittens neurones developed unconventional receptive fields which contained two and sometimes even three distinct excitatory regions (Singer & Tretter, 1976b). The distance between these discharge centers was on the order of 10 deg and corresponded to the spacing of the stripes in the grating which the kittens had previously been exposed to. The formation of such unconventional receptive fields can again be accounted for by selective stabilization of excitatory connections which have a high probability of being active in contingency with the postsynaptic target cell: In the striate cortex of visually inexperienced cats the excitatory regions of receptive fields are larger than in normal cats and on occasion subtend up to 20 deg. (Singer & Tretter, 1976a,b). The most likely substrate for such far reaching spread of excitation are axon collaterals of cortical pyramidal cells which run tangential to the cortical surface and can be traced over distances of several millimeters (Fisken et al., 1973; Szentagothai, 1975). As indicated schematically in Fig. 2.5 receptive fields with spatially separated discharge areas will form when the animal is exposed to a periodic pattern and when those intracortical connections stabilize selectively which interconnect neurones that tend to be activated simultaneously. With normal experience spatial relations between contours are of course much more variable and complex and as a consequence the experience dependent modifications of the intracortical associative collateral system can be expected to assume an extremely complex pattern, too. This could explain why the functional contribution of these abundant collaterals has so far escaped conventional receptive field analysis with simple stimuli.

The conclusion from this brief survey is that the experience-dependent modifications in the developing visual cortex can be accounted for by modification rules which formally resemble those proposed by Hebb (1949).

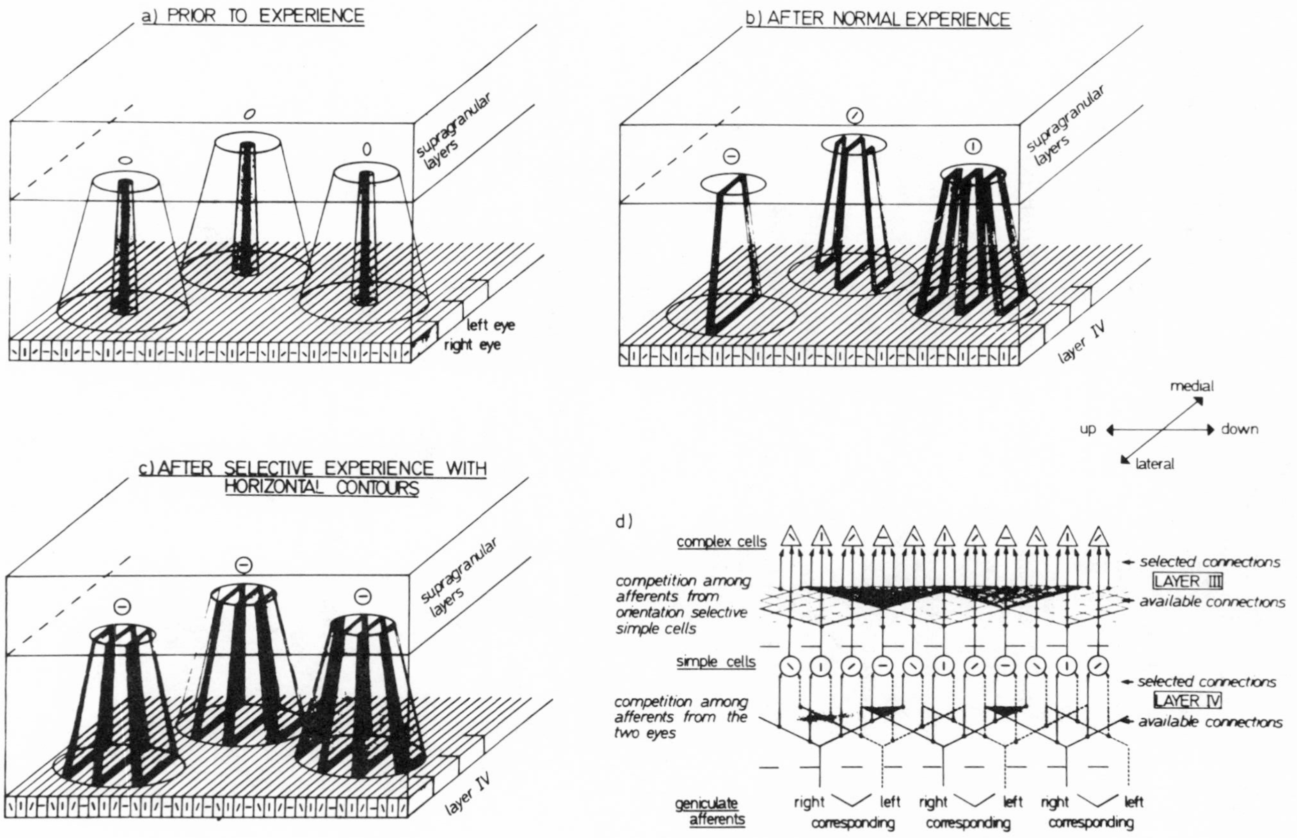
a) PRIOR TO EXPERIENCE
supragranular layers
left eye
right eye
b) AFTER NORMAL EXPERIENCE
supragranular layers
layer IV
medial
up
down
lateral
c) AFTER SELECTIVE EXPERIENCE WITH HORIZONTAL CONTOURS
supragranular layers
layer IV
d)
complex cells
competition among afferents from orientation selective simple cells
simple cells
competition among afferents from the two eyes
geniculate afferents
selected connections
LAYER III
available connections
selected connections
LAYER IV
available connections
right
left
corresponding
right
left
corresponding
right
left
corresponding

FIG. 2.4

Evidence for a Polymodal Control of Experience
Dependent Modifications

Several recent studies indicate that, in order to induce modifications of cortical functions, retinal signals do not only have to drive cortical cells — in which case it would suffice that they conform with the receptive field properties of striate cortex neurones — but they must in addition be adequate in the more global context of visuo-motor integration. Even when contour vision is unrestricted retinal signals may fail to induce modifications of cortical connectivity when the position or the motility of the eyes or the proprioceptive signals from the extraocular muscles are interfered with and abnormal.

We deprived kittens of vision in one eye by lid suture and simultaneously rotated the other open eye surgically within the orbit (Singer et al., 1979a; 1982a). This led to severe disturbances in visuo-motor coordination. As indicated by behavioral testing the kittens responded to these problems by developing a nearly complete neglect of visual stimuli rather than by modifying their central visuo-motor programs. Subsequent electrophysiological analysis revealed that the retinal signals from the open eye had failed to consolidate the pathways from this eye and had failed to induce competitive repression of the afferents from the deprived eye. Numerous cells had stopped responding to light stimuli altogether but a substantial fraction of the remaining cells continued to be binocular and excitable from both eyes. Thus, although retinal responses to contours were readily available and

---

FIG. 2.4   (*Opposite page*) Schematical representation of experience dependent selection of intracortical pathways relaying activity from prespecified orientation selective cells in layer IV onto second order cells in non-granular layers. It is assumed that prior to experience connections between first and second order cells are divergent and overlapping whereby coupling is strongest between first and second order cells within the same vertical cylinder (shaded columns in a) and decreases gradually with increasing tangential distance. With unrestricted experience (b) connections originating from first order cells sharing the same orientation preference are selectively consolidated at a particular second order cell. Because of their competitive advantage vertically ascending connections consolidate always and hence second order cells become selective for the same orientation as the first order cells located in the respective cylinder. In addition, however, second order cells maintain connections also with first order cells processing signals from adjacent visual field regions provided that they share the same orientation preference. Corresponding to the spatial organization of the receptive field of the second order cell sampling occurs along different vectors in the retinotopically organized matrix of first order cells. With restricted contour vision (c) only those connections between first and second order cells become consolidated which originate from first order cells capable of responding to the experienced orientation, the others become repressed by competition. Second order cells assume selectivity for the experienced orientation only. The schematical representation in (d) suggests that experience dependent modifications at the level of binocular convergence can be considered at least formally as similar to modifications in the domain of orientation selectivity.

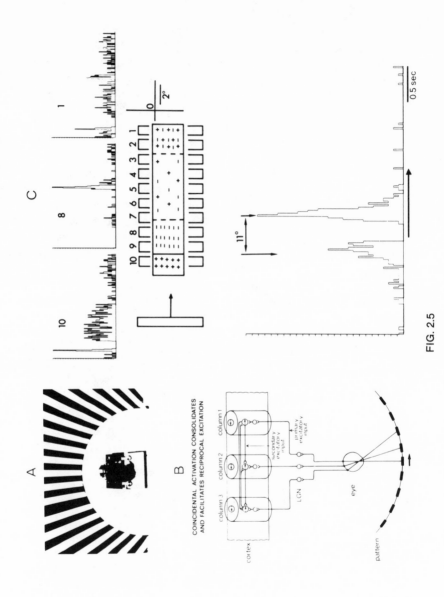

CONCIDENTIAL ACTIVATION CONSOLIDATES
AND FACILITATES RECIPROCAL EXCITATION

FIG. 2.5

although these activity patterns should have been suitable to drive cortical cells they failed to consolidate the connections with the open eye and at the same time failed to inactivate the afferents from the deprived eye (Fig. 2.6).

A similar result was obtained in kittens made strabismic by surgically deviating both eyes (Singer et al., 1979b). These kittens split in two populations. The larger group developed alternating fixation and used either of the two eyes but only one at a time for fixation and visual guidance. The other group appeared to have difficulties overcoming the bilateral misalignment of the eyes and failed to appropriately use either of the eyes. Visual behavior remained poor in both eyes. In the former group, as one expects from strabismic kittens, the large majority of cortical cells had become monocular, roughly equal portions responding exclusively either to the ipsi- or to the contralateral eye. By contrast, in the second group the majority of cortical cells had remained binocular. Competitive repression of the respective non-dominant eye had failed to occur despite the incongruency of retinal signals conveyed by the two eyes. A very similar finding has recently been reported by Crewther et al. (1980) for kittens in which both eyes were deviated by cyclotorsion. Also in this preparation retinal signals from the two eyes are incongruent but nonetheless a substantial fraction of cortical neurones had remained binocular. These results suggested that experience dependent modifications are gated by additional, non-retinal signals.

FIG. 2.5   (*Opposite page*) Paradigm for selective consolidation of pathways between neurones processing activity from spatially distant areas in the visual field. A: Exposure condition allowing for repeated and contingent activation of the subset of cortical neurones that have vertically-oriented RFs and are located in projection columns whose retinotopic relation matches the spatial distance of the stripes. B: Schematic representation of the interactions between contingently activated neurones. For the selected subset of cortical neurones with vertically oriented RFs and adequate retinotopic correspondence, activity in the reciprocal intercolumnar excitatory collaterals is contingent upon activation resulting from direct subcortical input. If selection among excitatory pathways is gated by a matching process between pre- and postsynaptic activity, such contingency should result in selective consolidation of interactions between simultaneously-driven neurones. This in turn should lead to RFs with several, spatially distant, excitatory areas, one resulting from direct subcortical input, the others from selectively-consolidated intercolumnar pathways. C: Example of a RF with two, spatially separated excitatory regions from a supragranular cell in the visual cortex of a cat exposed according to the paradigm in (A). The histogram at the bottom shows the response to a vertically-oriented slit of light that slowly moved from the periphery of the visual field towards the vertical meridian. The RF consists of two discharge areas separated by 11°. This distance corresponds to the spatial frequency of the grating used during exposure. Both excitatory regions could be mapped with stationary stimuli. Stimulus positions 1–11, and the location of the RF relative to the area centralis, are represented in the schematic drawing. As indicated by the selected histograms of responses to the stationary flashed stimuli, mixed on/off responses were obtained from the medial excitatory region, and spatially separated on/off responses were obtained from the lateral region. (From Singer, 1979a).

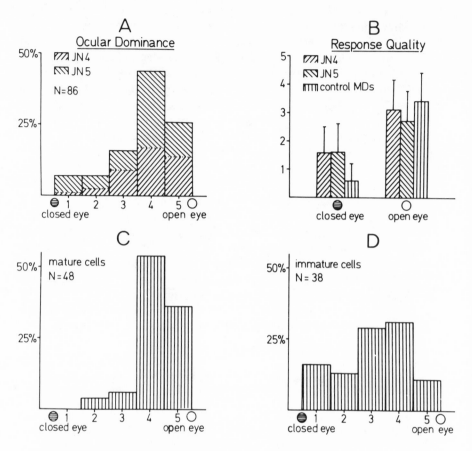

FIG. 2.6 a) Ocular dominance (OD) distribution (dark columns) of striate cortex neurones of six kittens raised with one eye closed and the open eye rotated. The hatched columns refer to the percentage of cells excitable from the two eyes in relation to the total
sample of analysed cells (N = 375). The horizontal broken line indicates the percentage
of light-reactive cells. Classes 1 and 5 comprise monocular cells responding exclusively to
either the right (deprived) or the left (normal) eye. Classes 2 and 4 refer to binocular cells
in which one eye is dominant. Class 3 contains cells responding equally to both eyes. Note
the symmetry of the OD distribution and the low percentage of light reactive neurones.
b) Average indices for the quality of responses obtained from the two eyes. In normal cats
these values range from 3.4 to 3.8.
c) OD distributions for cells with sluggish (hatched columns) and vigorous (blank columns) responses. Note the bias towards the open rotated eye in the OD distribution of vigorously responding cells.
d) OD distribution of non-oriented cells (hatched columns) and percentage of non-
oriented cells among neurones in the respective OD classes (blank columns). Cells lacking
orientation selectivity are dominated by the deprived eye. (From Singer, Tretter and
Yinon, 1982a).

A first indication for one of the sources of such permissive signals came from experiments in which we tested the effect of abolishing the proprioceptive signals that are generated by the stretch receptors of the extraocular muscles (Buisseret & Singer, 1983). We interrupted proprioception in dark-reared five-week-old kittens by severing bilaterally the ophthalmic branches of the trigeminal nerves. In addition we either sutured closed one eye or induced strabismus by resecting the lateral rectus muscle of one eye. Subsequently, the kittens were raised in normally lighted colony rooms and investigated with electrophysiological methods after they had passed the critical period. In case modifications had occurred in response to the altered retinal signals the large majority of cortical cells should have become monocular by that time and should respond to the only open eye in the monocularly deprived kittens or to either the ipsi- or the contralateral eye in the strabismic kittens. However, in both groups we found the majority of cells still binocular which suggests that proprioceptive signals from extraocular muscles are involved in gating experience dependent modifications of cortical connectivity (Fig. 2.7). In addition to the non-occurrence of competitive interactions between afferents from the two eyes we found also a number of abnormalities in other receptive field properties. Since these abnormalities were present also in the other kittens in which retinal signals failed to induce modifications and since these abnormalities are important for the interpretation of mechanisms they will be dealt with in a later chapter.

Evidence for a Control of Experience Dependent Modifications by Non-Specific Modulatory Systems

The kittens in which retinal signals failed to induce changes in cortical connectivity had in common to attend less to visual stimuli than normal kittens. In order to determine whether this was secondary to impaired maturation of visual cortex functioning or whether the deficit in visual attention was the cause of impaired maturation, a visual neglect syndrome was produced by placing lesions in the medial thalamus of kittens (Singer, 1982). Subsequently, we determined whether this sensory neglect led to impairment of experience dependent consolidation of cortical functions. In five-week-old dark-reared kittens the splenium of the corpus callosum was split to allow access to the third ventricle and then a small lesion was placed in the intralaminar nuclear complex of one hemisphere. Simultaneously one eye was sutured closed with the goal of using changes in ocular dominance as an indicator for experience dependent modifications. As in adult cats (Orem et al., 1973) these lesions led to a contralateral sensory hemineglect. When visual stimuli were presented simultaneously in both hemifields the kittens would consistently neglect the stimulus in the hemifield contralateral to the lesion

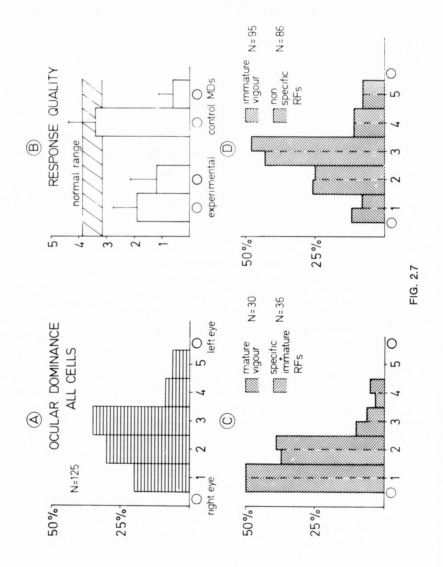

FIG. 2.7

50

and orient towards the other target. Similarly, acoustic stimuli or somatic stimuli close to the midline elicited orienting responses that were nearly always directed towards the side contralateral to the normal hemisphere. After the kittens had grown up for at least three more months in normally lighted colony rooms the receptive fields of single cells were investigated in the visual cortex of the two hemispheres. In areas 17 and 18 of the normal hemispheres conditions were identical to those obtained with conventional monocular deprivation. By contrast, in the hemisphere containing the lesion the majority of the cells had remained binocular showing only a slight bias in the ocular dominance distribution towards the open eye (Fig. 2.8). Thus, although both hemispheres had received exactly the same signals from the only open eye, these signals induced modifications only in the normal hemisphere but remained ineffective in the hemisphere which — because of the lesion — "attended" less to retinal stimulation. In this hemisphere also other parameters such as responsiveness to light and selectivity for stimulus orientation were abnormal indicating that retinal signals had not only failed to induce competitive suppression of the deprived afferents but had also failed to support the development or consolidation of normal receptive field properties.

Another significant abnormality of the hemisphere containing the lesion became apparent when during the experiment we tried to raise cortical excitability with electrical stimulation of the mesencephalic reticular formation. In normal animals this stimulus produces a large surface negative field potential over the visual cortex of both hemispheres and a massive facilitation of thalamic and cortical transmission (for review see Singer, 1977b; 1979b). In the kittens with the thalamic lesion these effects were greatly attenuated in the hemisphere containing the lesion while they were fully developed in the other. Thus, the thalamic lesion had obviously affected modulatory systems known to control thalamic and cortical excitability as a function of arousal and per-

---

FIG. 2.7   (*Opposite page*) Ocular dominance distributions of three kittens in which the left eye was closed by lid suture and in which proprioceptive signals from extraocular muscles were disrupted by bilateral section of the ophthalmic branch of the fifth cranial nerve. The ocular dominance histogram A reflects a moderate bias towards the open right eye but contrary to the condition after conventional monocular deprivation the majority of the neurones continue to respond to stimulation of both eyes. As indicated in B, the average indices for the vigour of responses to optimally aligned light stimuli are lower for the normal eye than in cats with conventional monocular deprivation or in totally normal cats (hatched range). As expected from the persistence of binocular cells the corresponding indices for responses from the deprived eye are higher in the experimental kittens than in the control MDs. In histogram (C) ocular dominance is plotted separately for cells responding vigorously to light and possessing normal or close to normal orientation selectivity; in histogram D ocular dominance is plotted of cells with immature response vigour and non-selective receptive fields. The ocular dominance distribution of the former is markedly biased towards the open eye while it remained virtually symmetrical for the latter. (From Buisseret and Singer, 1981).

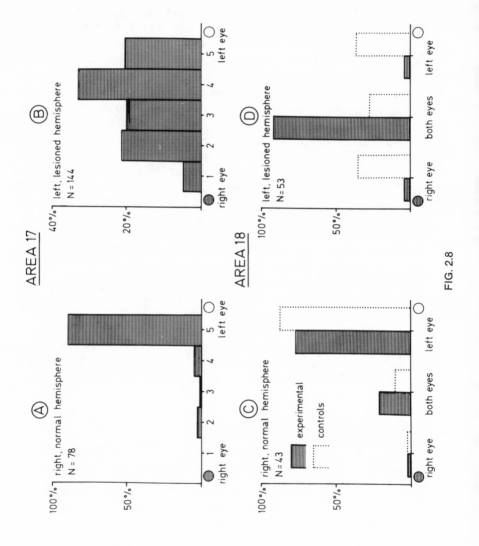

FIG. 2.8

52

haps also selective attention. This agrees with the behavioural evidence that the lesion had actually produced deficits in attention and supports the notion that modulatory systems might be involved in the control of cortical plasticity and act as a permissive gate.

Accepting this interpretation it was to be expected that electrical activation of the centrencephalic modulatory systems might facilitate experience dependent modifications of cortical functioning. It is well established that despite prolonged and intensive retinal stimulation modifications cannot be produced in the visual cortex of anesthetized and paralyzed kittens (Buisseret et al., 1978; Freeman & Bonds, 1979; Singer, 1979b). Thus, the expectancy was that substituting facilitatory influences of modulatory systems by electrical stimulation of the mesencephalic reticular formation or of the intralaminar thalamic nuclei might bring about modifications despite anesthesia and paralysis.

Five-week-old dark-reared kittens were prepared as is usual for acute electrophysiological experiments. They were anesthetized with nitrous oxide supplemented by barbiturates and paralyzed with a muscle relaxant. Several hours after the end of surgery we started to stimulate one eye with a slowly moving star pattern, the other eye remained closed. As expected, this procedure never led to changes in ocular dominance even when light stimulation was continued over two to three days. However, in 9 out of 10 kittens, in which the light stimulus was paired with brief electrical stimulation of either the reticular formation or the medial thalamus, clear changes in ocular dominance towards the open, stimulated eye became apparent after one night of monocular conditioning (Singer and Rauschecker, 1982). These changes were seen at the level of evoked potentials elicited either with phase reversing gratings or with electrical stimulation of the optic nerves and they were also apparent at the level of single unit receptive fields (Fig. 2.9). Moreover, there

---

FIG. 2.8   (*Opposite page*) The effect of unilateral thalamic lesions on developmental plasticity. Ocular dominance (OD) distributions in area 17 (A,B) and 18 (C,D) of the normal hemisphere (A,C) and of the hemisphere containing the lesion (B,D). Ocular dominance in the striate cortex was assessed from PSTH analysis of single unit receptive fields. In the hemisphere containing the lesion numerous cells have remained binocular despite monocular deprivation while in the other hemisphere ocular dominance had changed as expected from monocular deprivation. In area 18 ocular dominance was determined from single unit responses to electrical stimulation of the two optic nerves. To allow comparison with control data (columns drawn with dotted outlines) from monocularly deprived cats three classes were formed comprising cells responding to the right nerve alone, the left nerve alone, or both nerves. In area 18 the effects of conventional monocular deprivation are less pronounced in the hemisphere contralateral to the deprived eye than in the ipsilateral hemispheres (columns drawn with dotted outlines in D). However, in the hemisphere containing the lesion many more cells remained binocular than in the control cats, while in the normal hemisphere the shift in ocular dominance is similar to the shift in the corresponding hemisphere of the controls. (From Singer, 1982).

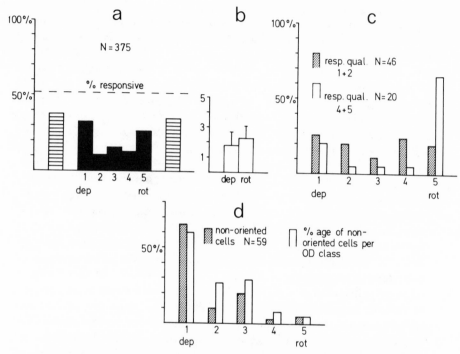

FIG. 2.9 Ocular dominance distributions (A,C,D) and average indices for the vigour of responses (B) of single cells recorded from striate cortex of two kittens which had 18 hrs of conditioning monocular light stimulation paired with electrical stimulation of medial thalamus prior to single unit analysis. Cells in ocular dominance classes 1 and 5 responded exclusively either to the ipsilateral closed eye or to the contralateral conditioned eye. Cells in class 3 reacted equally well to stimulation of either eye and cells in classes 2 and 4 responded more vigorously to one of the two eyes. The distribution in A summarizes the ocular dominance of all responsive cells in the two kittens In4 and In5. It shows a clear bias in favour of the conditioned eye although 67% of the cells are still binocular. The average vigour of responses from this eye has attained nearly the same level as responses from the normal eye in cats raised with conventional monocular deprivation, while the vigour of responses from the deprived eye is abnormally low but not yet as poor as that of responses from the deprived eye in conventional MDs (B). The distribution in C shows the ocular dominance of cells whose response vigour was ≥ 3 and whose orientation selectivity was in the normal range while the distribution in D summarizes the remaining cells in which either property was rated abnormal. This comparison reveals that the bias in the total sample of cells (A) is essentially caused by cells which have attained normal response properties. (From Singer, 1982).

was an indication from both evoked potential and single unit analysis that the gain of excitatory transmission in the pathways from the conditioned eye had increased and that cortical cells had become more selective for contrast gradients and stimulus orientation. These results are in line with the issue of the lesion experiments and further corroborate the hypothesis that non-specific modulatory systems which increase cortical excitability facilitate cortical plasticity.

Covariance Between Ocular Dominance Changes, Neuronal Responsiveness and Receptive Field Specificity

With conventional monocular deprivation nearly all neurones in striate cortex stop responding to the deprived eye but responsiveness and receptive field specificity are found normal when tested through the experienced eye. In the preparations described in the preceding paragraphs numerous cells maintained connections with both eyes despite monocular experience or strabismus. Whenever this was the case, the vigour of responses to optimally aligned light stimuli and the selectivity for stimulus orientation were found to be abnormally low in a substantial fraction of cells. Thus, retinal signals have not only failed to suppress the afferents from the deprived eye but they have also failed to increase the gain in pathways of the normal eye and to guide the development of normal receptive field selectivity. This suggested that the three parameters might depend on the same developmental process and if such were the case they should covary. Correlation analysis confirmed this expectancy. Cells were subdivided into different groups according to the vigour of their responses and the selectivity of their receptive fields. This revealed that the ocular dominance distributions of cells rated as immature on either or both of these scales had by and large the same symmetrical shape as that found at the beginning of the critical period. The fraction of cells rated as mature, by contrast, did reflect the influence of visual experience (Figs. 2.6, 2.7). In the monocularly deprived cats the ocular dominance distribution of mature cells showed a bias towards the open eye and in the strabismic cats it showed the familiar u-shaped distribution with a substantial bias in favour of the respective contralateral eye. Moreover, among these mature cells those with simple receptive fields were disproportionally numerous. Since the fraction of "mature" cells was always very low, never exceeding 20%, their biased distribution had, however, never substantially distorted the ocular dominance distribution of the whole cell sample. This was different in the kittens in which ocular dominance changes were successfully induced by combined retinal and brain stimulation. Also here, the immature cells maintained an essentially symmetrical ocular dominance distribution but the fraction of mature cells had increased to more than 50% after 18 hours of monocular stimulation. These cells had a marked bias in their ocular dominance towards the stimulated eye and since they were numerous they effectively distorted the ocular dominance distribution of the whole cell sample (Fig. 2.9).

These correlations suggest that the same processes which lead to ocular dominance changes are also improving excitatory transmission and receptive field specificity. This is in agreement with the previous suggestion that variations of all three parameters might be based on similar processes. All experimental results could thus be accounted for by the single assumption that the extent to which experience dependent modifications have occurred along the afferent connections to individual neurones was variable. When the changes in response to retinal stimulation were substantial the cells changed their ocular dominance, became well excitable by the dominant eye and acquired mature selectivity for stimulus orientation. When activity dependent modifications did not occur the cells maintained their original connectivity and immature receptive fields.

An exception appears to be certain neurones with simple receptive fields. Nearly in all the kittens with exclusive monocular experience we encountered several monocular cells with mature response properties which were driven by the deprived eye. These cells had always simple receptive fields and were usually encountered in the hemisphere contralateral to the deprived eye. In agreement with the findings of Fregnac and Imbert (1978) this indicates that a certain population of cells can develop normal receptive field properties even when the eye to which these cells are connected was deprived of contour vision. Since monocular cells with simple receptive field properties are preferentially located within layer IV (Gilbert, 1977) this relates also well to the results of the deoxyglucose study (Singer et al., 1981): they have indicated that cells in layer IV are capable of developing preferences for stimulus orientations which have never been experienced. It thus appears as if certain cortical cells — and this is the large majority — would require experience dependent modifications of their initial connectivity to acquire mature receptive fields while others — most likely certain simple cells at the input stage — do not. The former are usually binocular and maintain modifiable connections with the two eyes while the latter tend to be monocular from the beginning and do not change ocular dominance.

A Voltage Dependent Threshold for Experience Dependent Modifications?

The evidence presented so far indicates that in a variety of conditions retinal signals fail to induce modifications even though they are eliciting responses in cortical cells. Thus, temporal contingency between pre- and postsynaptic activity appears to be only a necessary but not a sufficient condition for the occurrence of adaptive changes. Additional "now print"-signals appear to be required and these seem to be available only when retinal signals are attended to and identified as appropriate in a behavioural context.

Although we are far from understanding the neuronal mechanisms of experience dependent modifications I would like to propose a concept which requires only one additional assumption in order to account for the experimental results. This assumption is that the adaptive mechanism has a threshold, the critical parameter being the depolarization of the postsynaptic dendrite. Thus, changes in synaptic gain would occur only when dendritic depolarization trespasses a critical level. The occurrence of modifications does then depend not only on the activity of the specific afferents but also on the functional state of numerous other converging pathways which modulate the membrane potential of dendrites. As summarized in Fig. 2.10 these additional input systems can be subdivided into three major groups which exert an increasingly global control of dendritic depolarization: First, the large number of recurrent collaterals which spread tangentially in striate cortex; second, the numerous cortico-cortical connections which originate in other cortical areas and terminate on the dendrites of cells in area 17; and third, the non-specific afferents which ascend from subcortical structures and exert a modulatory control of cortical excitability. The extent to which a retinal signal depolarizes the dendrites of a particular cortical cell is thus dependent on a large number of matching operations occurring simultaneously in numer-

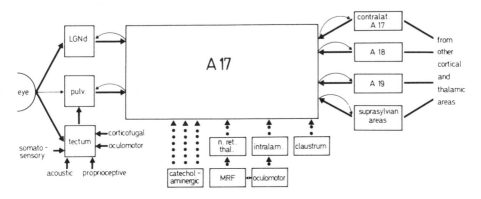

Afferent systems to striate cortex potentially capable of exerting channel specific (——) and global (•••) control of resonance

FIG. 2.10   Schematical representation of projection systems supposed to gate experience dependent modifications in striate cortex. Both feedback loops between processing areas and modulatory "non-specific" systems determine the excitability of neurones in visual cortex. The probability that retinal signals induce modifications of cortical connectivity would thus depend both on polymodal matching operations and on the internal state of the brain.

ous distributed but interconnected neurones. In order to elicit maximal resonance in a cortical neurone the retinal signal would not only have to match the receptive field properties of this neurone but would have to be appropriate also with respect to the response properties of numerous other cells. Part of these cells are located in the same cortical area but may be selective for other features of the stimulus than the cell under consideration or may even process signals from more remote retinal areas. Other cells are located in different cortical areas and may no longer be purely visual but may receive input also from other sensory or even from motor systems. Apart from the stimulus configuration and its contextual relation with other sensory signals or ongoing motor activities excitation of these recurrent loops will of course depend to a critical extent also on the functional state of the "non-specific" modulatory systems and hence on behavioural states such as arousal and attention.

In agreement with the experimental results modifications in response to retinal signals are thus expected to occur only when these signals are appropriate not only with respect to the receptive field properties of striate cortex neurones but also with respect to cross-modal sensory processing and visuomotor coordination. But even if these conditions are in principle fulfilled it is required in addition that the retinal signals are received by an aroused brain and are actually attended to. The finding that reticular and thalamic stimulation facilitated cortical modifications despite the fact that the kitten had no behavioural control over the stimulus is not contradicting this interpretation. It should make no difference whether supracritical dendritic depolarization results from a global and diffuse increase of activity in a large number of converging afferents — as is probably the case with electrical activation of modulatory systems — or whether it results from selective activation of particular feed-back loops — as is probably the case in the behaving animal. A voltage dependent threshold of plasticity could thus serve as the final common path for the control of experience dependent modifications. No separate gating system would be required for the generation of a permissive "now print"-signal. The ensembles of distributed but interconnected nerve cells which process sensory signals and generate behavioural responses would act themselves as the gating system. Hence, the criterion for the "now print" decision would be set by the response characteristics of a very large ensemble of interconnected and cooperating nerve cells.

Such a distributed but non-global gating is consistent with the experimental results. They indicated a certain channel specificity of the gating process since in all preparations retinal signals had induced modifications in the connectivity of some cells but not of others. Channel specific control of experience dependent maturation of cortical functions is suggested also by psychophysical evidence. In strabismic humans who suffer from amblyopia it could be demonstrated that the development of cortical functions depends on retinal eccentricity. Visual functions such as spatial resolution and binocular integration may fail to develop normally in one part of the visual field — usually a region close to the projection of the fovea of the deviating eye — while they may be completely normal in adjacent regions (Sireteanu & Fronius, 1981; Sireteanu et al., 1981). This evidence for channel specific control of plasticity is of course compatible with additional global gating systems which could control plasticity simultaneously in all cortical areas such as have been postulated by Kety (1970). Kasamatsu and Pettigrew (1976, 1979) and Kasamatsu et al. (1979) provided evidence that changes in ocular dominance occur only if the concentration of cortical norepinephrine is sufficiently high. This is strong indication for a global control of cortical plasticity by the widely distributed norepinephrinergic pathways that ascend from locus coeruleus.

The notion that experience dependent modifications are gated does not reduce the validity of the classical Hebbian rules: Temporal contingency between pre- and postsynaptic activity is probably still the crucial parameter. To satisfy the experimental results we are forced, however, to postulate an additional parameter which is in turn dependent on the functional state of numerous other brain systems. As discussed above a voltage dependent threshold process in the postsynaptic dendrite could serve as such an additional parameter in that it could effectively gate modifications as a function of the actual state of the brain. Preliminary results on stimulus induced changes of extracellular Ca^{++} concentrations suggest that such a voltage dependent process might in fact exist. When light stimuli are coincident with electrical activation of the non-specific activating system — a condition sufficient to induce cortical modifications — sudden decreases of the extracellular Ca^{++} concentration can be observed. It is tempting to speculate that this reflects the action of voltage dependent Ca^{++} channels which enable Ca^{++} ions to enter into dendrites when a certain level of activation is trespassed. Much recent evidence is in fact suggesting that electrogenic Ca^{++} mechanisms exist in dendrites of vertebrate neurons and are particularly important during early development (for a review see Llinas, 1979). Accumulation of intracellular Ca^{++} could then in turn act as a permissive signal for the modification of synaptic efficiency (for a review see Kretsinger, 1979).

CONCLUDING REMARKS

Since experience dependent modifications of neuronal connectivity appear to be such a general feature of the developing visual cortex it appears appropriate to briefly speculate on their functional role in normal development. In general these processes have an associative function in that they selectively stabilize connections between those neurones which have a high probability of being active simultaneously. This has different consequences at different levels of cortical processing.

At the level where afferents from the two eyes converge such a selection could assure that only those afferents become consolidated which come from corresponding retinal loci in the two eyes. When the kitten is fixating targets with both eyes these afferents will convey very similar activity patterns and hence become stabilized selectively. This simple process could thus help to establish the extremely high precision in the connectivity between the two eyes and common cortical target cells that is required for binocular visual functions. Apart from the fact that it would be rather uneconomical to leave this specification to genetic instructions alone it appears indeed unlikely that such precision could be achieved without relying in addition on functional criteria. Retinal correspondence is dependent on factors such as the position of the eyes in the orbit or the interocular distance and these parameters are in turn subject to epigenetic modifications. It appears very unlikely, therefore, that precise correspondence of binocular connectivity can be established without relying on functional criteria for final specification. However, such selection according to functions can only be successful when the selection processes are gated as proposed above. Selection should only occur when the kitten is actually fixating a target with both eyes and it should not occur in all the many other instances in which the images on the two retinae are out of register because the eyes are not properly aligned. Experience dependent modifications occurring during these latter conditions would lead to competition between the afferents from the two eyes and to disruption of binocularity.

As mentioned briefly experience dependent modifications in the domain of orientation selectivity could assure that second order cells receive excitatory input only from those first order cells which share the same orientation preference. Two considerations indicate that this selection problem is again not a trivial one: Second order cells with large receptive fields have to receive input from numerous first order cells that may be distributed over several hypercolumns (Albus, 1975a,b; Hubel and Wiesel, 1974). Because first order cells sharing the same orientation preference are clustered within discrete regularly spaced columns this implies discontinuous sampling from clusters of first order cells which may be several millimeters apart. Moreover, because of the retinotopic organization of striate cortex, second order cells with elongated vertical receptive fields must receive input from first order cells along the longitudinal axis of striate cortex while second order cells with elongated horizontal fields must integrate input from first order cells along the mediolateral axis. Because of the continuity of contours in the natural environment this extremely complex specification of connections can again be achieved by selectively consolidating connections which have a high probability of being activated simultaneously. This selection is aided by the strong inhibitory interactions between cells with differing orientation preferences (Blakemore & Tobin, 1972) since this inhibition effectively prevents simultaneous firing of cells in columns with different orientation preferences. The finding that orientation selectivity of cortical neurones could remain immature even though retinal responses to oriented contours were readily available indicates that this selection process, too, is gated and probably occurring only when the pattern is sufficiently unambiguous.

The functional role of modifications at the level of the tangential intracortical connections is still unclear. With normal experience the combinatory complexity of possible contingencies becomes so exceedingly large that it is impossible to predict the resulting pattern of differentially weighted interactions. Again it can be expected that cells become associated preferentially which have a high probability of responding simultaneously in the presence of particular feature combinations. Such preferential coupling would enhance and prolong by reverberation the responses of distinct cell assemblies to particular, frequently occurring patterns. This would distinguish cells of the assembly from other neurones which are not able to join or to form a cooperating ensemble. These latter cells, too, will respond to stimuli containing the appropriate trigger features but if the combination of features does not match a previously established pattern of selective interactions, the responses of individual cells remain independent and will not be sustained by reciprocal facilitation. Experience dependent modifications at this level of cortical processing could thus be a first step towards the formation of cooperative cell assemblies whose coherent and reverberating responses would signal the presence of a particular previously experienced combination of features.

It thus appears that the experience dependent modifications of neuronal connectivity during early development share a number of features thought to be characteristic also of adult learning. Sensory signals lead to selective associations of neurones with distinct functional properties and as in adult learning the formation of such associations requires the active participation of the brain. Both the developing and the mature brain have the option to screen the continuous stream of afferent signals and to enable only those activity patterns to induce long lasting changes of neuronal interactions that have been identified as relevant in a global behavioural context. It is tempting to infer from these formal similarities between developmental plasticity and adult learning that both might depend on the same mechanism. Recent experiments in adult cats have in fact indicated that experience dependent changes of similar nature can occur in striate cortex even after the end of the classical critical period when manipulations of sensory signals force the animals to develop compensatory strategies (Singer et al., 1982b).

These changes, at least phenomenologically, resemble those occurring durng early development. The main difference is, that inactivation of neuronal transmission is fully reversible when it occurs after the end of the critical period while it is irreversible when it occurs during the critical period. This suggests that it is perhaps not so much the occurrence of modifications per se which is unique to the critical period but rather a developmental process which first provides an excess supply of connections by continuous proliferation of new contacts and second, permanently removes connections which had been losers in experience dependent modifications. Once these developmental processes terminate only the degrees of freedom for modification would become less but modifications of excitatory transmission are apparently still possible.

REFERENCES

Albus, K. A quantitative study of the projection area of the central and the paracentral visual field in area 17 of the cat. I. The precision of the topography. *Exp. Brain Res., 24,* 159–179 (1975a).

Albus, K. A quantitative study of the projection area of the central and the paracentral visual field in area 17 of the cat. II. The spatial organization of the orientation domain. *Exp. Brain Res., 24,* 181–202 (1975b).

Blakemore, C., & Tobin, E. A. Lateral inhibition between orientation detectors in the cat's visual cortex. *Exp. Brain Res., 15,* 439–440 (1972).

Blakemore, C., & VanSluyters, R. C. Reversal of the physiological effects of monocular deprivation in kittens: further evidence for a sensitive period. *J. Physiol. (Lond.), 237,* 195–216 (1974).

Blakemore, C., & VanSluyters, R. C. Experimental analysis of amblyopia and strabismus. *Brit. J. Ophthal. 58,* 176–182 (1974).

Blakemore, C., VanSluyters, R. C., Peck, C. K., & Hein, A. Development of cat visual cortex following rotation of one eye. *Nature, 257,* 584–586 (1975).

Buisseret, P., & Imbert, M. Visual cortical cells: their developmental properties in normal and dark reared kittens. *J. Physiol. (Lond.), 255,* 511–525 (1976).

Buisseret, P., Gary-Bobo, E., & Imbert, M. Ocular motility and recovery of orientational properties of visual cortical neurones in dark-reared kittens. *Nature, 272,* 816–817 (1978).

Buisseret, P., & Singer, W. Proprioceptive signals from extraocular muscles gate experience-dependent modifications of receptive fields in the kitten visual cortex. *Exp. Brain Res., 51,* 443–450 (1983).

Crewther, S. G., Crewther, D. P., Peck, C. K., & Pettigrew, J. D. Visual cortical effects of rearing cats with monocular or binocular cyclotorsion. *J. Neurophysiol., 44,* 97–118 (1980).

Cynader, M., Lepore, F., & Guillemot, J. P. Interhemispheric competition during postnatal development. *Soc. Neurosci. Abstr., 6,* 171.6 (1980).

Fisken, R. A., Garey, L. J., & Powell, T. P. S. Patterns of degeneration after intrinsic lesions of the visual cortex (Area 17) of the monkey. *Brain Res., 53,* 208–213 (1973).

Freeman, R. D., & Bonds, A. B. Cortical plasticity in monocularly deprived immobilized kittens depends on eye movement. *Science, 206,* 1093–1095 (1979).

Fregnac, Y., & Imbert, M. Early development of visual cortical cells in normal and dark-reared kittens: relationship between orientation selectivity and ocular dominance. *J. Physiol. (Lond.), 278,* 27–44 (1978).

Gilbert, C. D. Laminar differences in receptive field properties of cells in cat primary visual cortex. *J. Physiol. (Lond.), 268,* 391–421 (1977).

Hebb, D. O. *The organization of behaviour.* New York: Wiley, 1949.

Hubel, D. H., & Wiesel, T. N. Receptive fields, binocular interaction and functional architecture in the cat's visual cortex. *J. Physiol. (Lond.), 160,* 106–154 (1962).

Hubel, D. H., & Wiesel, T. N. Receptive fields of cells in striate cortex of very young, visually inexperienced kittens. *J. Neurophysiol., 26,* 994–1002 (1963).

Hubel, D. H., & Wiesel, T. N. Binocular interaction in striate cortex of kittens reared with artificial squint. *J. Neurophysiol., 28,* 1041–1059 (1965).

Hubel, D. H., & Wiesel, T. N. Uniformity of monkey striate cortex: A parallel relationship between field size, scatter and magnification factor. *J. Comp. Neurol., 158,* 295–306 (1974).

Hubel, D. H., Wiesel, T. N., & LeVay, S. Plasticity of ocular dominance columns in monkey striate cortex. *Phil. Trans. Roy. Soc. Lond. B., 278,* 377–409 (1977).

Imbert, M., & Buisseret, P. Receptive field characteristics and plastic properties of visual cortical cells in kittens reared with or without visual experience. *Exp. Brain Res., 22,* 25–36 (1975).

Kasamatsu, T., & Pettigrew, J. D. Depletion of brain catecholamines: failure of ocular dominance shift after monocular occlusion in kittens. *Science, 194,* 206–209 (1976).

Kasamatsu, T., & Pettigrew, J. D. Preservation of binocularity after monocular deprivation in the striate cortex of kittens treated with 6-hydroxydopamine. *J. Comp. Neurol., 185,* 139–162 (1979).

Kasamatsu, T., Pettigrew, J. D., & Ary, M. Restoration of visual cortical plasticity by local microperfusion of norepinephrine. *J. Comp. Neurol., 185,* 163–181 (1979).

Kety, S. S. The biogenic amines in the central nervous system: Their possible roles in arousal, emotion, and learning. In *The neurosciences, second study program.* F. O. Schmitt (ed.), pp. 324–336. New York: Rockefeller Univ. Press, 1970.

Kretsinger, R. M. The informational role of calcium in the cytosol. *Adv. in Cycl. Nucleotide Res., 11,* 1–26 (1979).

Llinas, R. The role of calcium in neuronal function. In: *The neurosciences, fourth study program.* F. O. Schmitt, & F. G. Worden (eds.), pp. 555–571. Cambridge, Mass: MIT Press, 1979.

Mitzdorf, U., & Singer, W. Monocular activation of visual cortex in normal and monocularly deprived cats: an analysis of evoked potentials. *J. Physiol. (Lond.), 304,* 203–220 (1980).

Orem, J., Schlag-Rey, N., & Schlag, J. Unilateral visual neglect and thalamic intralaminar lesions in the cat. *Exp. Neurol., 40,* 784–797 (1973).

Rauschecker, J. P., & Singer, W. Changes in the circuitry of the kitten's visual cortex are gated by postsynaptic activity. *Nature, 280,* 58–60 (1979).

Rauschecker, J. P., & Singer, W. The effects of early visual experience on the cat's visual cortex and their possible explanation by Hebb synapses. *J. Physiol. (Lond.), 310,* 215–239 (1981).

Sherk, H., & Stryker, M. P. Quantitative study of cortical orientation selectivity in visually inexperienced kittens. *J. Neurophysiol., 39,* 63–70 (1976).

Singer, W. Modification of orientation and direction selectivity of cortical cells in kittens with monocular vision. *Brain Res., 118,* 460–468 (1976).

Singer, W. Control of thalamic transmission by corticofugal and ascending reticular pathways in the visual system. *Physiol. Rev., 57,* 386–420 (1977). (a)

Singer, W. Effects of monocular deprivation on excitatory and inhibitory pathways in cat striate cortex. *Exp. Brain Res., 30,* 25–41 (1977). (b)

Singer, W. The role of matching operations between pre- and postsynaptic activity in experience-dependent modifications of visual cortex functions. In: *Neural growth and differentiation.* E. Meisami, & M. A. B. Brazier (eds.), pp. 295–310. New York: Raven Press, 1979. (a)

Singer, W. Central-core control of visual cortex functions. In: *The neurosciences, fourth study program.* F. O. Schmitt, & F. G. Worden (eds.), pp. 1093–1109. Cambridge, MA: MIT Press, 1979. (b)

Singer, W. Plasticity in the developing visual cortex depends on diencephalic structures mediating selective attention. *Nature,* (submitted) (1981a).

Singer, W. Central core control of developmental plasticity in the kitten visual cortex: I. Diencephalic lesions. *Exp. Brain Res., 47,* 209–222 (1982).

Singer, W., & Tretter, F. Receptive-field properties and neuronal connectivity in striate and parastriate cortex of contour-deprived cats. *J. Neurophysiol., 39,* 613–630 (1976). (a)

Singer, W., & Tretter, F. Unusually large receptive fields in cats with restricted visual experience. *Exp. Brain Res., 26,* 171–184 (1976). (b)

Singer, W., & Rauschecker, J. P. Central core control of developmental plasticity in the kitten visual cortex: II Electrical activation of mesencephalic and diencephalic projections. *Exp. Brain Res., 47,* 223–233 (1982).

Singer, W., Rauschecker, J., & Werth, R. The effect of monocular exposure to temporal contrasts on ocular dominance in kittens. *Brain Res., 134,* 568–572 (1977).

Singer, W., Yinon, U., & Tretter, F. Inverted monocular vision prevents ocular dominance shift in kittens and impairs the functional state of visual cortex in adult cats. *Brain Res., 164,* 294–299 (1979). (a)

Singer, W., von Grunau, M., & Rauschecker, J. Requirements for the disruption of binocularity in the visual cortex of strabismic kittens. *Brain Res., 171,* 536–540 (1979). (b)

Singer, W., Freeman, B., & Rauschecker, J. Restriction of visual experience to a single orientation affects the organization or orientation columns in cat visual cortex: A study with Deoxyglucose. *Exp. Brain Res., 41,* 199–215 (1981).

Singer, W., Tretter, F., & Yinon, U. Central gating of developmental plasticity in kitten visual cortex. *J. Physiol. (Lond.), 324,* 221–237 (1982). (a)

Singer, W., Tretter, F., & Yinon, U. Evidence for long term functional plasticity in the visual cortex of adult cats. *J. Physiol. (Lond.), 324,* 239–248 (1982). (b)

Sireteanu, R., Fronius, M., & Singer, W. Binocular interaction in the peripheral visual field of humans with strabismic and anisometropic amblyopia. *Vision Res., 21,* 1065–1074 (1981).

Sireteanu, R., & Fronius, M. Naso-temporal asymmetries in human amblyopia: consequence of long-term interocular suppression. *Vision Res., 21,* 1055–1063 (1981).

Szentagothai, J. The module concept in cerebral cortex architecture. *Brain Res., 95,* 475–496 (1975).

Wiesel, T. N., & Hubel, D. H. Extent of recovery from the effects of visual deprivation in kittens. *J. Neurophysiol., 28,* 1060–1072 (1965).

Wolfe, J. M., & Owens, D. A. Evidence for separable binocular processes differentially affected by artifically induced anisometropia. *Am. J. Optom. and Physiol. Optics, 56,* 279–284 (1979).

Yinon, U. Eye rotation in developing kittens: The effect on ocular dominance and receptive field organization of cortical neurons. *Exp. Brain Res., 24,* 215–218 (1975).

3 Monday's Discussion

Cooper: What we shall try to do today and after the succeeding luncheons is to open up for discussion what the speakers have said during the conference. I think that we will have many questions that haven't been answered during the talks themselves; perhaps some of these questions will be answered here.

Chip, maybe you could explain the experiment in which you had the four conditions. I got lost there. Is it explainable?

Levy: The point of the experiment was to activate distinct regions of the dendrites which were separated by about 100–200 microns. The data showed that the interaction generated by the powerful input, the permissive event for change (whether it be potentiation or depotentiation), was localized in the dendritic region where the synapses were active and did not spread the 100 or 200 microns to the other synapses. In other words, this permissive event did not spread down the dendrite.

Sherman: Your data really represent population spikes or some population potential. In order to interpret it that way, you have to know that each individual dendritic tree has all of these synapses on it. Is that known?

Levy: Well, I could just give you some numbers and tell you that each dendrite has only a small fraction of the total projection, but the reason that the experiments worked so well was that we were looking at many, many cells and at a naturally averaged experiment. At any one time, I don't know if I'm recording from 100 or 10,000 cells. We assume that, with these field potentials, the system has averaged things out for us and that, on the average, some fraction of the input is going to every cell. When we did current-source density measurements, the specificity was much greater than we had ever imagined. Our current-source density maps go down to 7.5 micron separations.

Sherman: If some cells receive inputs only on their peripheral dendrites and others only on their proximal dendrites, then you wouldn't expect any interactions.

Levy: Yes, but I would never expect a cell like that, because there are spines all over all the cells' dendrites, so I don't think it's numerically a very likely situation. It's theoretically possible, but it just doesn't seem to be likely.

Singer: I think the important advantage of this preparation is that single cells can be studied. I recently had a conversation with Per Andersen, asking him specifically about the contribution of coincidental postsynaptic spiking as a permissive signal. Clearly it isn't; he had recorded from the cells, preventing them from responding to the conditioning presynaptic volley. This didn't abolish potentiation at all, indicating that the processes must be localized presynaptically or within the dendrites. It's still unclear whether it's a pre- or postsynaptic process that causes this increase.

Levy: Our data say it's both. Our anatomy data indicate very strongly that the synapses have increased in number and in size with potentiation.

Changeux: How can you count the synapses? When you say the number of synapses have increased, what do these numbers mean?

Levy: I should describe the experimental setup. We condition one ipsilateral system at high frequency, and the other ipsilateral system is either unconditioned or stimulated at a low frequency that does not induce potentiation. Then the comparisons are made between hippocampi so that we have an internally matched, controlled experiment each time we do an animal; the data always compare one side with the other. These matched differences are averaged across animals to see if we have an effect.

Changeux: Isn't that by electron microscopy and by thin sections?

Levy: Yes.

Changeux: And you count what? Contours?

Levy: We identify synapses by the standard criteria of postsynaptic density and presynaptic aggregation of synaptic vesicles. We then draw the postsynaptic densities and the spine heads, and we measure everything we can think of measuring. The measurements are stereologically corrected as suggested by Underwood (*Quantitative Stereology,* New York: Addison-Wesley, 1970), and the assumptions involved in this correction have been confirmed in serial sections.

Crick: Since you're comparing two sides of the same animal, you have a built-in control, so that should be all right. But what one really wants to know is the magnitude of the synaptic changes and the number of synapses comparable with the effects you see.

Levy: I don't know how to scale it. I don't know what fraction of the total number of synapses I'm activating, so I don't know what change I'm really dealing with.

Crick: But can't you make a crude estimate to see if you're in the right ball park?

Levy: I haven't been able to.

Chapman: How good is the spatial resolution that you get from the field potentials?

Levy: If you use a small electrode, less than 20 microns is possible. That's why we had to go to shorter and shorter distances between recording sites for our current source densities.

Castellucci: You have segregation of the input; do you look at the whole postsynaptic cell, the whole dendritic tree? If you have segregation of input and only one input is potentiated, you would expect to have some spines being modified on the same cell. Do you test for that?

Levy: Let me see if I understand your question: If we have potentiation, we should also have depotentiation. Is that what you mean?

Castellucci: No. You have an input and you potentiate that input. You look at the spines on the postsynaptic cells. Now, I think that the anatomy tells you that there is segregation, namely, that one part receives the input and the other part doesn't. Most of the change is there, but did you have regional change? The way you presented it, it seems that everything was changed.

Levy: If you remember, the graph that showed ΔN_A had a staircase effect with various levels till you got to the center level, and then ΔN_A went negative. That center region is the region of greatest activation, but the region where there are fewer synapses after conditioning. But the total length of active membrane, if we call the postsynaptic density the active membrane, is unchanged. So we claim that these results represent both potentiation and depotentiation happening in one region — fewer synapses but larger synapses. In regions right next to the central region, we had our largest absolute increases in synapses and integrated active membrane — the amount of postsynaptic density. We have to postulate that sprouting has occurred a very short distance away from the central region of conditioning, forming new synapses a little further along the dendritic axis. It will obviously require two or three more experiments to prove a hypothesis like this, but that's the hypothesis we're working on now.

Crick: Can I summarize by saying that, where you expected to find the change, either you did or they were next door. Is that what you're saying?

Levy: In terms of number, yes. But there were changes everywhere.

Daniels: Chip, I wonder if you could say more about the paired contra- and ipsilateral stimulation — how much greater was the paired response than the sum of the two alone?

Levy: We should have given you the electronic subtraction so that you could appreciate that more easily. However, there is no single answer, since, as you go through the wave form, there's progressively more and more depolarization and the nonlinear effect increases.

Daniels: What was the nonlinear effect?

Levy: The theoretical summation of the two wave forms is greater than the actual . . . .

Daniels: Was it twice as great as the summation?

Levy: It depends on how I turn my stimulator.

Singer: But when you have synapses close together, wouldn't there always necessarily be a shunting of the input, so that whatever happens depends to a crucial extent on the geometry?

Levy: Yes.

Pettigrew: Editor's note: At this point the recording is rather noisy. In essence Pettigrew points out that Lynch's laboratory reported changes in the number of shaft synapses following long-term potentiation in CA1 of the hippocampus. He raises the point that they may have observed synaptogenesis or more likely an intraconversion from spine synapses to shaft synapses. Such an intraconversion might only require a "contractile mechanism" rather than "active growth."

Castellucci: In contrast to Levy's work using the entorhinal projection to the dentate gyrus, the ultrastructural correlates in CA1 have an ambiguity. Here one cannot be sure that the observed changes are at synapses that are even part of the Schaffer–CA1 system.

Levy: I agree. We don't know if those "new" synapses are on the CA1 pyramidal cell that is generating most of the electricity. These new shaft synapses could be formed by or with an interneuron either de novo or from intraconversion. By the way our work in the dentate replicates this change in shaft synapses. When we look at the shaft synapse category, we have nearly a doubling on the conditioned side compared to the control side. But the shaft synapses are less than 5% of the total. This is also true in CA1. That's why Lynch is unable to conclude whether there is a change in the absolute number of total synapses or not.

Pettigrew: Yes, but who knows what the contribution of the spine synapse is? It might be quite ineffective. Who knows what sort of dendritic integration is going on?

Levy: That's true. Absolutely.

Crick: Why do you say it's ineffective, Jack? It may be, but only if it's different. It isn't because of the spine.

Edelman: Are the diameters of the dendritic shaft constant?

Levy: This is a critical question. Rall's hypothesis for the spine stem controlling the electrotonic conduction of the synaptic event into the dendrite is one of the best hypotheses for explaining the neurophysiological effects. It does make a lot of sense. We've been doing some serial section work, but we've completed only one animal. So far we've only been able to analyze 20% to 30% of the synapses. We think there are changes of spine stems, but it's very hard research.

Donahue: Did you see changes in the spine head sizes?

Levy: Yes; they were shown on the graphs.

Donahue: Okay. With what can you compare the changes you found? Fifkova didn't show an increase in absolute number of synapses.

Levy: No, she didn't. But, in general, I don't care to compare my data with Fifkova's because she doesn't use appropriate stimulation frequencies and doesn't measure the neurophysiological effects. She stimulates at 15 Hz; that's a frequency we find ineffective for inducing long-term potentiation, but quite effective for inducing afterdischarges.

Crick: What sort of change did you get in the spine head?

Levy: Again, it depends on what region you look at. In the region of primary activation, there were many large spine heads, but in the border regions, there were more small spine heads. The increased number of small spine heads is what you would expect if there were an intraconversion of large to small or if there were growth of new synapses.

Crick: How much larger does "large" mean? Do you mean 20% larger, or 50% larger, or 100% larger in volume or surface?

Levy: Probably about 30%. It's so substantial that experienced observers can look at both sides in the electron microscope, and guess which one got the stimulation. By the way, we don't score our data that way, we take the photographs, shuffle them together, and give them to someone else who doesn't know anything about the situation.

Castellucci: In your analysis, you assume that the potentiation is a change in the excitation. But what happens if you have just an IPSP that is becoming more effective or less effective? That will increase the drive on the postsynaptic cell.

Levy: I believe that our data are very clear in ruling out inhibitory synapses as causing the long-term potentiation because we can detect potentiation at the earliest onset times of the postsynaptic response, far too soon to be affected by an inhibitory loop. On the other hand, I do think that we have to pay attention to inhibitory loops because we know they're going on. And I believe that I can make a claim for the nonphysiological nature of the ipsi–contra/medial–lateral experiment (the experiment with four conditioning electrodes) because we know we're inducing tremendous amounts of inhibition during these conditioning trains. The inhibition is going to come on about 2 msec after the onset of the excitation. In the hippocampus, we always speak in the Ecclesian sense of the inhibitory synapses being only on the soma and doing their inhibiting down there, even though we know from the binding studies of Palacios, Young, and Kuhar (*Proceedings of the National Academy of Science*, 1980, *77*, 670–674) and from the neurochemical studies (Nadler et al., *Brain Research*, 1974, *79*, 465–475; *Brain Research*, 1977, *131*, 241–258) looking at the distribution of GABA and GAD in the molecular layer, that there must be inhibitory synapses distributed throughout the molecular layer. So I'd like to propose that we are inducing inhibition throughout the dendrite, but we're sculpting that inhibition away with the powerful afferents that we're stimulating. That's the possible artifact of the localized dendritic domains. In the normal animal, you won't stimulate all at once 10,000 fibers that originate in a single region of the entorhinal cortex. I would expect that you would have firing throughout the entorhinal cortex, phased over time and space, so that you would have a very phased, gentle type of excitation throughout the neuron. You won't find the amount of inhibition in a behaving animal that you do in an experimental situation.

Crick: Could you be a bit more explicit as to why it's not inhibition? I didn't understand that word "sculpting."

Levy: I'm saying that the whole cell is inhibited, and potentiation is going to take place in the region where the excitatory synapses are really active, but their effect for potentiation/depotentiation doesn't spread because of the pervasive inhibition.

Crick: So there's a balance between excitation and inhibition: Locally the excitation wins, and further away the inhibition wins. Is that what you're saying?

Levy: But I'm not going to do an experiment to prove it.

Castellucci: But even natural conditions are likely to include nuclei from other systems. The site of maximum excitation is the site of maximum inhibition. The reason why the excitation is winning is that it arrived just a little bit before the inhibition. Thus, under natural stimulation, you may have a lot of inhibition where the excitation is, and the balance could be modified. I'm not sure we can rule that out at this time.

Crick: Is it really true that there is anatomical evidence for wide distribution of Type 2 synapses over the whole length of the dendrites? In other systems, they are often concentrated either in the center or in the proximal part of the dendrite.

Levy: Are you asking about the ultrastructural evidence for inhibitory synapses? That doesn't exist in the dentate. I'm relying on neurochemical data to claim that there are inhibitory synapses.

Ebner: Our work with the turtle cortex says inhibitory synapses shouldn't be ruled out. It seems unfortunate to count them out just because they're only 10% of the total population in that system. They certainly respond to thalamocortical input when it is stimulated or removed.

Levy: One of the pressing experimental questions is to figure out a way of doing some of these same experiments with an inhibitory system. Why should we waste all the inhibitory synapses as just being part of a passive feedback modulating circuit? They should also have an elemental learning rule. I interpret Rutledge's undercut cortex data as showing that inhibitory synapses can change as an effect of stimulation. So there is evidence that inhibitory synapses can be modulated.

Rutledge: Did you see any changes in the concentration of the presynaptic vesicle populations in these cells? Did you look for them?

Levy: We're just starting to quantify the presynaptic elements because of our growth hypothesis. What we have to show is clear. If we're going to claim there are new synapses, we have to show that there are also more presynaptic structures.

There are interesting kinds of new synapses and there are new synapses that aren't as interesting. If you have an afferent going to a postsynaptic cell and then that afferent grows another synapse with that postsynaptic cell, that would probably be equivalent to just changes of synaptic efficacy. But if you have an afferent not going to this cell, and then growing a synapse with that cell, that would seem to be a different order of synaptic growth. And that is a very, very difficult experimental question to get at. I don't know how to do it.

Cooper: Could you go over your discussion of the new time sequences? You were trying to see whether the correlation between pre- and post- could have time delays.

Levy: It works only in one direction.

Cooper: Could you just remind me what that direction was.

Levy: The weak conditioning stimulus had to come before the strong one. It's just the opposite of what we predicted before the experiment.

Cooper: That's a good kind of experiment to have. So you're saying that, in order for it to be effective, the presynaptic input has to come before the postsynaptic response.

Levy: Well, it's always best when they come together.

Arbib: I'd like to raise a general question. I had thought that everyone had agreed that there was no possibility of there being Hebb synapses, and then this person comes along and says, "Hey! I've found one."

Cooper: When did everyone agree on that?

Levy: I agreed 4 years ago.

Arbib: I wondered if, for some of the people who've thought about this, you'd perhaps say something about why they had become convinced that there weren't Hebb synapses. I think that most experimentalists have come to feel that they'd been looking for evidence for Hebb synapses and that they hadn't seen them. Stent came up with a model of a Hebbian synapse that was felt to be a totally ad hoc and farfetched model. In the last few years it seems that theorists have still been modeling Hebb synapses, while experimentalists have been quite convinced that there weren't any. Maybe Vincent could say whether he agrees with my perception.

Castellucci: No. People began to find some non-Hebbian phenomena, so the focus was there and the analysis was pursued in that direction—for example, in the work I did with Bob Wurtz. However, that was a negative experiment. I think other people in other systems tried briefly and found no strong effect. But the theory as such was not rejected.

Crick: Wouldn't you argue that it depends on frequency and intensity? That if you don't get that right, you won't see it?

Levy: Actually, Bliss and Lømo (*Journal of Physiology,* 1973, *232,* 357–374) did the proper experiment; they varied intensity. The experiment didn't work. As a matter of fact, according to Goddard (personal communication), Bliss and Lømo couldn't do long-term potentiation a year after their study came out. They started using the wrong frequencies, and they started going to lower and lower frequencies. That's why there's a big lag in the work in LTP for a while. They knew enough to do the experiment — a lot of people knew enough to do the experiment. It's just that there were many instances of the intensity experiments not working. It's a question of knowing where to go to show it.

Cooper: I'd like to make a comment about that. If there is evidence for a type of synaptic modification, one can't be sure that's the only kind that exists. I would guess that there exist a whole variety of modifications that are related by a few basic physiological mechanisms. My personal belief is that there's absolutely no reason why the rule for the modification must be entirely of the Hebbian type. I think it's much more likely that we'll find a variety of rules, of which only some will be Hebbian or variations of Hebbian.

Cowan: I don't really understand the point that you're making about the Hebb synapse. What evidence do you have that would rule out the possibility that what you have is simply presynaptic facilitation — but in a network? Because all you're doing is recording population averages? How can you possibly say that you have evidence for correlated pre- and postsynaptic activity at the individual junctions?

Levy: Well, the activity's correlated because we make it correlated. You don't believe that?

Cowan: No. You're presenting population averages all the time. You're not recording intracellularly from single cells, are you?

Levy: I may be recording from 10,000 cells.

Cowan: Well, then, how can you say anything about what goes on locally?

Levy: Somewhere things are going on together. We showed convergence.

Cowan: Yes, but in a population where you have 10,000 cells, particularly when you know you've got some cooperativity there, you cannot say anything about the local mechanism or change, just because you have coincidence in time and possibly even in space.

Cooper: I think, Jack, that what you're saying is that there is another way to explain his data. And the answer is "No doubt there is." However, what he shows is that, if you do have a correlation between the pre- and post-, then you get an effect, and one very simple and straightforward way of explaining that effect is to assume a Hebb-type modification. It's certainly not the only way to explain it.

Cowan: I thought the purpose of doing scientific research at this level is to try to exclude many hypotheses.

Cooper: No experiment has ever been done that cannot be explained by a variety of hypotheses.

Cowan: Well, then, I would claim that none of these experiments excludes simple facilitation in networks. There isn't a single experiment that shows definitely the existence of the notion that Hebb synapses exist.

Cooper: Well, now, I think you have to be careful.

Cowan: Show me how you can exclude it.

Cooper: If you say that you can explain his data with another theory, it's incumbent upon you to construct that theory.

Cowan: It's trivial to construct a theory that will account for that with nonlinear facilitation in a network.

Edelman: I believe that it was Demerec who once said, when he was asked how he interpreted his experiments, "First, we try with the data, and then we try without the data."

Rutledge: But, Jack, these are monosynaptic systems he's working with. The changes were seen exceedingly early.

Cowan: Some years ago, Ben Burns and Bliss and Uttley produced a piece of work which they claimed demonstrated the existence of Hebb synapses by potentiation experiments. I took their data and spent a week going over it, using exactly the methods they had in their paper. All I could produce from it was that the presynaptic stimulus facilitated the pathway. There was absolutely no evidence for Hebbian synapses in their work, even though they had a monosynaptic pathway and population averages.

Castellucci: Actually, there may be a big difference between the non-associative type of learning and synaptic modification and the associative type. Perhaps within a few years from now, we'll be in a position to test that. Terry Walters and Carew and Kandel have found correlates in the motor neuron that execute a program. At present, there is nothing new known about the associative mechanism and what's going on — whether it is a presynaptic phenomenon or a postsynaptic phenomenon. It may be that it's Hebbian. We don't know.

Cowan: Again, I think one has to very careful. Some years ago, I thought I had some fairly sharp evidence for the existence of Hebbian-type synapses in connection with the phenomenon of visual adaptation to sine-wave gratings. I learned an interesting lesson there. If you assume you're dealing with a single mechanism at each point in the visual field, then you assume a single homogeneous population of cells. If you try to make a model with that kind of system of adaptation to a grating of a particular spatial frequency, to a specific number of cycles per degree of visual angle, then you need a Hebb synapse mechanism to account for the experimental data. However, as soon as you realize that there may be more than one mechanism at each point in the visual field, then you have, not a homogeneous population, but three to five populations with slightly different spatial scales, coupled nonlinearly: then simple fatigue is all you need to account for the experimental data. In fact, in every situation in which you have a homogeneous population and you need some kind of cooperativity to store things in, you can always accomplish the same thing with pure, simple facilitation in a system of more than one population with nonlinear coupling.

Cooper: Yes, but you have to couple the output neurons to each other.

Cowan: Therefore, I do not see any alternative to intracellular techniques for getting anywhere close to what is going on in a single synapse.

Cooper: Well, you have to make your assumptions clear. In order to explain his data without a Hebbian-type rule, you have to have interactions between the outgoing neurons of a very nonlinear type.

Cowan: Not *very* nonlinear.

Cooper: All right, but still a nonlinear type.

Editor's note: Tape is noisy at this point. Castellucci apparently asks for evidence against some disinhibitory phenomenon to account for potentiation.

Levy: At a phenomenological level, I think the data and the anatomy of the system are very good. Vince, we're talking about 1.8 msec, and you say that it's going to produce presynaptic inhibition?

Castellucci: No, you may have reduction of inhibition, but not presynaptic inhibition.

Levy: Why would that change excitatory current flow of the conditioned afferents but not the unconditioned afferents?

Cowan: I'd like to ask you a question that Ivar Giaever asked Gary Lynch when he presented similar material last year. At the levels of current density that you employ, how do you know you're not just burning holes in the hippocampus and just producing injury discharges?

Levy: Injury discharges are a very specific phenomenon. We do not get injury discharges. As far as burning holes is concerned, we know we're using aphysiological stimuli, but how can potentiation be explained by burning holes at the stimulation site?

Cowan: What sort of current densities are you using in the stimuli?

Levy: I don't know, but it does not detract from the controls that we do to show that the cooperative phenomenon has gone on.

Cowan: You can get cooperativity in epilepsy when there are focal lesions.

Levy: I'll have to take your word for the kind of cooperativity that is.

Cowan: It is cooperativity.

Crick: Jack, have you answered the criticism that this is all done in a very short period of time?

Cowan: The reason I think it might be an injury discharge is that it does occur within a very short time.

Levy: We can wait a day. We can test a day later.

Cowan: Yes, that's what Gary said, too.

Crick: But more to the point, the change is reversible.

Levy: Yes. Moreover, the same "high" current density produced by ipsilateral conditioning stimulation produces both the potentiation or the depotentiation of crossed system.

Crick: Then that's the point. It's not just an injury discharge.

Cooper: I think that, before you say that you can explain his data with some system of nonlinear coupling, you have to look at all the data—the going up, the going down, the reversibility.

Cowan: I was just trying to sharpen the question. It seems to me that, before you can say that you have a Hebb mechanism, you have to be able to record at a local level.

Cooper: What he's saying is that he has a phenomenon and that it can be explained simply by assuming a Hebbian mechanism. That does not show that the Hebbian mechanism exists.

Cowan: Well, I claim that I can explain it just as simply with facilitation.

Singer: There are conditions where you can't get away with presynaptic processes only—for instance, in the visual system, the result of monocular deprivation gives a clear indication for the participation of postsynaptic mechanisms. One subset of afferent pathways is disconnected, not because it is deprived, but because the pathways from the open eye consolidate. Hence you have to make additional assumptions.

Cowan: Yes, but since he's recording from a population, there can be all sorts of feedbacks in the network that could provide the cooperativity. In other words, the actual synaptic modification may be purely presynaptic and you may have external feedbacks all over in the network. How can you rule that out?

Cooper: You cannot rule that out. The point is that he has some data, and this is a simple explanation of the data.

Cowan: I would claim it's consistent both with the equation that you've posited and with an infinity of other equations with slightly different assumptions about what's in the network.

Crick: How would you rule it out by putting an electrode into a single cell?

Cowan: If one could record intracellularly, pre- and postsynaptically, then one could see whether or not coincident stimulation and firing induced changes in the cell.

Singer: To be strict, you would have to isolate individual cells in your preparation.

Changeux: Editor's Note: At this point the tape is noisy. Apparently a question is asked about the strict correlation between postsynaptic activity and the induction of potentiation in the hippocampus.

Singer: It works without postsynaptic spikes?

Editor's note: There are two examples of potentiation in which the conditioning stimulation does not always produce a population spike. Preceding conditioning by a single commissural pulse is one. The other is conditioning the projection to the dentate originating in the far lateral entorhinal cortex.

Levy: Yes.

Singer: But this doesn't mean anything. Hebb's synapses would work as well with dendritic depolarization alone as the required postsynaptic signal. In principle, soma spikes are dispensable.

Crick: When you get a situation like this, you have to adopt the rule "Go round about, Peer Gynt." If it turned out, for example, that the necks of the spines were altered, which is, I think, clearly postsynaptic, that would at least move the argument to another level, and then we could think about molecular biology. I think you're right in principle, though I doubt if you're correct in fact. But I also think the answer will have to come by looking at another technique.

Cowan: But even if the spines changed, that would not rule out presynaptic facilitation.

Crick: Well, it would show that something was happening postsynaptically.

Levy: An intracellular experiment could prove the postsynaptic locus of the decision process. There is an experiment that someone's going to do in a couple of years that would obviously be done best in the granule cells' mossy fibers to CA3. There's a problem with all these intracellular recordings; you're at an electrotonic distance away from your synapses. In CA1, it's pretty bad. It's very hard to reverse Schaffer collateral synaptic potentials in CA1, so you're pretty far away, far enough away so that your experiment is not going to be very good. But in the mossy-fiber system you can get reversal potentials for the excitatory input because they are right next to the cell body. You could voltage-clamp while you are conditioning the mossy input. And if that blocked conditioning, or if you injected EDTA and that blocked conditioning, then you have the experiment. So it's theoretically possible and someone will probably do the experiments in the next couple of years.

Cowan: I used an equation very similar to the one you put up, and it's very important to know whether that really is true or whether it's just another one of these mysterious theoretical devices that we like to use because they're so beautiful and do so many things.

Cooper: Well, Jack, I think that perhaps that subject will be elucidated to a certain extent tomorrow morning.

4
Some Constraints Operating on the Synaptic Modifications Underlying Binocular Competition in the Developing Visual Cortex

J. D. Pettigrew
National Vision Research Institute of Australia

In this chapter I deal with two independent lines of investigation on the process of binocular competition that takes place in the visual cortex, particularly during early development. The first follows on from the experiments begun by Wiesel and Hubel (1965) using alternating monocular deprivation to examine the degree of synchrony of afferents from each eye that is necessary for the maintenance of binocularity. Our extension and variation of these experiments lead us to conclude that the process of synaptic modification underlying binocular competition is akin to the processes postulated by Hebb (1949), because a conjunction of both presynaptic and postsynaptic activity appears to be necessary for modification to occur. In addition, our results lead to the counterintuitive conclusion that a large degree of asynchrony, of the order of some seconds, is tolerated by the synaptic modification process (Blasdel & Pettigrew, 1979).

This last result, implying a certain degree of "sloppiness" in the time domain, is hard to reconcile with the fact that the binocular, disparity-selective neurons forming the basis for stereoscopic vision have very fine tolerances in the time domain. Moreover, these very fine tolerances on the part of disparity-selective neurons appear to improve during the early neonatal period, when one might expect that the large tolerance for asynchrony would lead to a gradual degradation in the face of the high degree of modifiability of binocular connections and the noise injected into the system by the imprecision of binocular coordination of eye movements in the young animal. These problems could be overcome if there were a mechanism, independent of the visual system, that could regulate plasticity in such a way that synaptic modification only took place in the presence of stable eye position. I propose that the pontine nucleus, locus coeruleus, could subserve such a role, and the second series of experiments deals with the possibility that this nucleus may be able to regulate synaptic plasticity in the visual cortex.

Binocular Competition and Hebb's Rule

Hebb's rule (1949) that synaptic modification takes place if firing at a given synapse is associated with firing at other synapses, seems very likely to apply to the synaptic modification processes underlying binocular competition, as there are a number of situations where binocular competition can be shown to occur only when there is a conjunction of presynaptic and postsynaptic activity. As already pointed out by Stent (1973) this would be an effective way to implement Hebb's rule because in most cases the firing of a number of associated synapses will be necessary to drive the postsynaptic cell. Demonstrations that firing of a postsynaptic cortical cell is necessary for modification in synaptic terminals of geniculate afferents has already been provided at this meeting by the work of Singer (Chapter 2). A third demonstration that the firing of a cortical neuron is necessary before synaptic modification takes place, and that therefore the process may be thought of as Hebbian, is provided by the experimental arrangement illustrated in Fig. 4.1.

In this experiment we take advantage of the orientation selectivity of individual cortical neurons to examine the effects of asynchronous stimulation of the afferent pathways from each eye. The kitten, raised normally to the age of 4 weeks, is now exposed to rotating gratings whose orientations are always 90° apart in the two eyes. Bearing in mind that cortical neurons are orientation selective, whereas neurons in the lateral geniculate nucleus providing afferents to the cortex are not, one can see that this mode of stimulation will have the following consequences: (1) the mean level of activity in lateral geniculate nucleus will not change as the gratings rotate; (2) cortical neurons will first be stimulated through afferents from one eye, and then as the gratings rotate, will be stimulated through afferents from the other eye; (3) the degree of asynchrony between driving from the geniculate afferents of the two eyes will vary as a function of the speed of rotation of the two gratings.

At the appropriate slow rate of rotation we found that binocularity broke down, and can thereby conclude that synaptic modification was not a result of activity in the geniculate afferents per se, but rather in the effective conjunction of geniculate activity with postsynaptic cortical cell driving. In addition, by varying the rate of rotation and looking at the consequent preservation or destruction of binocularity, we could examine the constraints operating upon this modification process in the time domain.

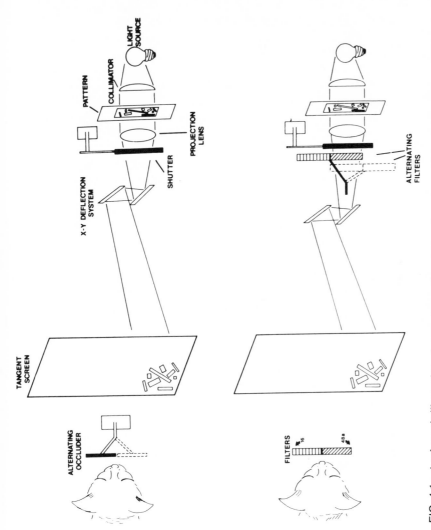

FIG. 4.1 A schematic illustration of apparatus used to alternately expose each eye to randomly oriented contours. The upper arrangement utilized occluders, and the lower utilized filters to optically achieve monocular stimulation and vary interonset times. A more complete description of apparatus appears in Blasdel and Pettigrew, 1979.

81

Timing Constraints upon Binocular Competition

There is a surprising tolerance of asynchrony in the afferent channels from the two eyes on the part of developing binocular cortical neurons. This is shown in Fig. 4.2. Binocularity appears to be quite normal when as much as 1 sec elapses between successive stimulation of afferent pathways from the two eyes, and binocularity is not reduced substantially until the interval approaches 10 secs. This suprising and counterintuitive result conjures up the picture of binocular competition in which bulbous terminals from each eye lugubriously compete for the available space on the surface of the postsynaptic neuron. A long time constant is supported by the results of other studies, and if one plots data available on the effect of different rates of alternating monocular deprivation, one comes up with Fig. 4.3. Here binocularity is seen to be a linear declining function of log interonset time where the time constant for a 50% reduction in binocularity lies somewhere between 10 and 100 secs.

Conflict Between Timing Requirement for Binocular Competition and for Stereoscopic Mechanisms

If we accept, for the present, the remarkable degree of asynchrony that appears to be tolerated by developing binocular connections, we are faced with a paradox. This paradox arises because the timing constraints operating on the mature stereoscopic visual system are stringent indeed. Stereoacuity in a cat is around a few minutes of arc (Mitchell, 1980; Pettigrew, Nikara, & Bishop, 1968) in the presence of eye movements producing a retinal image drift of around 4°/sec, so the adult system is clearly capable of detecting fractions of a msec. Because the developing binocular system of the cat is very malleable, and because a developing kitten is subjected to continually varying disparities because of variations in target distance and because of variations in its own disjunctive eye position, a tolerance on the part of the binocular mechanisms for such large time intervals ought inevitably to lead to degradation of the disparity-selective network. This does not occur. In fact it has been shown that disparity selectivity is gradually improved as a result of visual experience during development (Pettigrew, 1974). The system clearly needs another constraint that would limit synaptic modification to those times when the animal was stationary and its eyes were in steady binocular alignment. In other words, there should be a "gate" for synaptic plasticity, such that synaptic modifications are made possible only when there is independent information available from the motor system that there are no self-generated changes in disparity occurring.

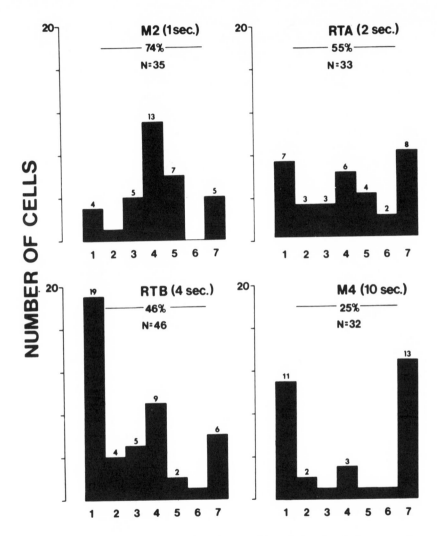

FIG. 4.2 The effect of interocular asynchrony on binocularity of cortical neurones. Ocular dominance distributions are shown for kittens reared in different asynchronous conditions: 1, 2, 4, and 10 seconds. Categories 1 and 7 are monocularly driven cells, and categories 2 to 6 are binocularly driven cells. The percentage of binocular cells and number of cells recorded are shown in upper portion of each histogram. Refer to Blasdel and Pettigrew (1979) for a more detailed description.

The Locus Coeruleus as a "Gate" for Synaptic Plasticity

The proposed gate should have two properties. One, it should have access to information about self-generated movements, particularly eye movements, that is independent of visual information, so that it may identify those periods of time when binocular disparity is not changing because of self-generated movements. Two, it should be capable of enabling or disabling the underlying mechanism of synaptic modification so that modifications of binocular connections do not take place when binocular disparity is being varied because of self-generated movements.

Although work in this area is still very much in its infancy, there are good reasons for proposing that the monoaminergic fiber systems might help play a role in these two functions. In particular, the nucleus locus coeruleus, whose cortical projections are noradrenergic, does seem to play a role in the

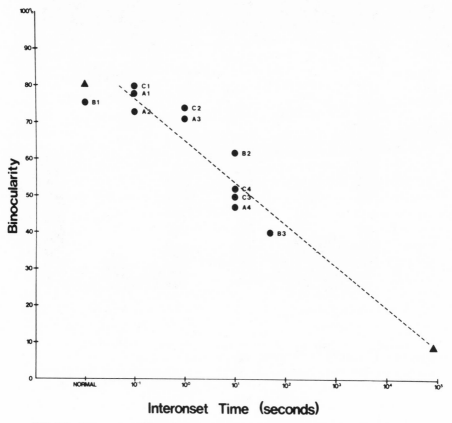

FIG. 4.3   Percentage of binocular cells as a function of interonset time. The abscissa is a log scale. For a more complete description see Blasdel and Pettigrew (1979).

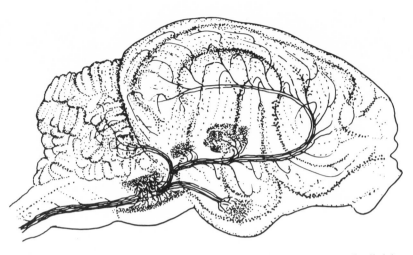

FIG. 4.4   The projections of the nucleus locus coerulus in cat. For a more detailed description, see Pettigrew (1982). (From Pettigrew, J. D., Pharmological control of cortical plasticity. *Retina,* 1982, *2*(4), p. 361.)

maintenance of cortical plasticity. A large number of experiments support this point of view (for example see Kasamatsu, 1980; Kasamatsu & Pettigrew, 1976; Kasamatsu, Pettigrew, & Ary, 1979; Pettigrew, 1978).

In summary it can be said that: (1) the widespread projections of the locus coeruleus to many cortical regions, and the diffuse distribution of axonal varicosities capable of releasing norepinephrine, many of which do not form classical synaptic specializations (Itakura, Kasamatsu, & Pettigrew, 1980) are consistent with the view that the system is involved in a regulatory role, which might include the regulation of synaptic plasticity. Figure 4.4 shows the schematic illustration of the diffuse axonal projection and distribution of the nucleus locus coeruleus; (2) depletion of cortical norepinephrine results in a loss of synaptic plasticity in the cortex of young kittens (Fig. 4.5); (3) replacement of depleted norepinephrines by local microperfusion results in a restoration of cortical plasticity (Pettigrew & Kasamatsu, 1978); (4) recovery of binocularity following a prior period of monocular deprivation can be accelerated by simultaneous perfusion of norepinephrine and retarded by depletion of norepinephrine. This last observation is important because it shows that norepinephrine can be associated with an increase or a decrease in binocularity according to the nature of the visual input. In other words, norepinephrine is associated with plastic change whether this involves an increase or a decrease in binocularity, and it can be regarded as having a general effect on synaptic plasticity rather than some specific pharmacological effect on the synaptic mechanism underlying a cortical function such as binocularity; and (5) adult animals, which do not normally show evidence of

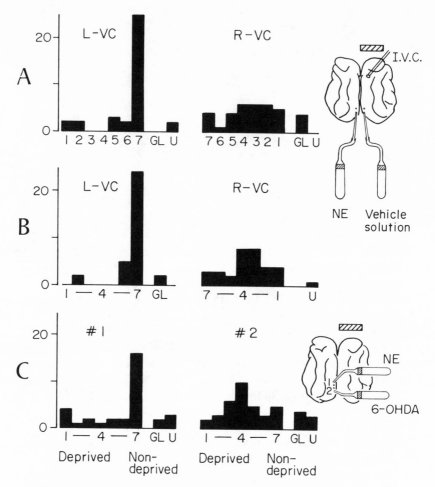

FIG. 4.5 Ocular dominance distributions for three monocularly deprived and catecholamine-depleted cats. The ocular dominance distributions shown on the left exhibit a shift in ocular dominance to the open, nondeprived eye. These regions were perfused with norepinephrine. The ocular dominance distributions on the right do not exhibit a shift to the open eye, and these recordings were made from regions depleted of catecholamines. For a more complete description of this figure and experiment, see Pettigrew and Kasamatsu (1978).

much cortical plasticity, can be induced to show synaptic modification by treatment with norepinephrine and by cyclic nucleotides (Kasamatsu, 1980; Kasamatsu et al., 1979).

REFERENCES

Blasdel, G., & Pettigrew, J. D. Degree of interocular synchrony required for the maintenance of binocularity in kitten's visual cortex. *Journal of Neurophysiology*, 1979, *42*, 1692–1710.

Hebb, D. O. *The organization of behavior*. New York: John Wiley & Sons, 1949.

Itakura, T., Kasamatsu, T., & Pettigrew, J. D. Catecholaminergic terminals in kitten visual cortex: Laminar distribution and ultrastructure. *Neuroscience, 6*(2), 159–176, 1981.

Kasamatsu, T. A possible role for cyclic nucleotides in plasticity of visual cortex. *Soc. Neurosci. Abst.*, 1980, *6*, 494.

Kasamatsu, T., Pettigrew, J. D., & Ary, M. Restoration of visual cortical plasticity by local microperfusion of norepinephrine in kittens and cats. *J. Comp. Neurol.*, 1979, *185*, 163–182.

Kasamatsu, T., Pettigrew, J. D., & Ary, M. Recovery from the effects of monocular deprivation: Acceleration by norepinephrine and retardation by 6-hydroxydopamine. *J. Neurophysiol.*, 1981, *45*(2), 254–266.

Pettigrew, J. D. The effect of visual experience on the development of stimulus specificity by kitten cortical neurons. *J. Physiol.* (London), 1974, *237*, 47–74.

Pettigrew, J. D. Is the locus coeruleus involved in cortical plasticity? *Trends in Neuroscience*, 1978, *1*, 73–74.

Pettigrew, J. D., & Kasamatsu, T. Local perfusion of norepinephrine maintains plasticity in visual cortex. *Nature*, 1978, *271*, 761–763.

Pettigrew, J. D., & Kasamatsu, T. Preservation of binocularity after monocular deprivation in the visual cortex of kittens treated with intraventricular 6-hydroxydopamine. *J. Comp. Neurol.*, 1979, *185*, 139–162.

Pettigrew, J. D., Nikara, T., & Bishop, P. O. Binocular interaction on single units of cat striate cortex: Simultaneous stimulation by single moving slit with receptive fields in correspondence. *Exp. Brain Res.*, 1968, *6*, 391–410.

Stent, G. S. A physiological mechanism for Hebb's postulate of learning. *Proc. Nat. Acad. Sci. USA*, 1973, *70*, 997–1001.

Wiesel, T. N., & Hubel, D. H. Comparison of the effects of unilateral and bilateral eye closure on cortical unit responses in kittens. *J. Neurophysiol.*, 1965, *28*, 1029–1040.

5 Remarks about the "Singularity" of Nerve Cells and its Ontogenesis

Jean-Pierre Changeux
Institut Pasteur
Paris, France

The word *complexity* is commonly found in any description of the functional organization of the nervous system. But, instead of covering our ignorance, it should be used as incentive to find rules that would facilitate its description and possibly shed some light on its genesis.

The topic of this chapter is limited to the fine anatomical organization of the nervous system. The complexity arising from nerve impulse coding, although essential for a complete understanding of higher brain functions, is not discussed.

Three rather simpleminded theoretical points are made about: (1) the level of organization at which diversity becomes large enough to create complexity; (2) gene expression and the ontogenetic development of connectivity between nerve cells; (3) one plausible mechanism that might create diversity from a small number of genes. Finally, experimental data relevant to these ideas are discussed.

THE COMPLEXITY OF THE FUNCTIONAL ORGANIZATION OF THE NERVOUS SYSTEM

The description of the organization of natural systems may hinge on two different kinds of complexity. One, which might be referred to as *unorganized complexity,* is that presented, for instance, by a suspension of bacteria, when one wishes to know the particular position, orientation, and movement of any one of the bacterial cells. The other, more relevant to the description of the anatomy of the nervous system and referred to as *organized complexity,* deals with relationships among elements of a system assumed to have a fixed position in time and space. The level of organization considered as useful to characterize the complexity of the nervous system is that of the neuron and its connections with other neuronal or nonneuronal cells of the organism.

The description of nerve cells and their mutual relationships has been investigated in the past by two distinct although complementary approaches. "Histological" techniques led to the description of neuronal morphology and of the local distribution of some biochemical and antigenic markers. "Microphysiological" techniques, thanks to the use of juxta- or intracellular electrodes, have defined the functional modalities of individually recorded cells.

The nervous system of vertebrates contains ensembles of cells that show the same general shape (soma, axonal, and dendritic arborizations), synthesize and release the same neurotransmitter, and contain the same receptors for neurotransmitters and various surface antigens. This is, for instance, the case for the Purkinje cells of the cerebellar cortex. Even if, in the near future, subgroups might be defined within the Purkinje cells, their number is expected to be small compared to the actual total number of Purkinje cells (which may reach $1-2 \times 10^7$ in man) (Palay & Chan-Palay, 1974).

Thus it appears legitimate to group within the same *category* the smallest ensemble of cells with the same morphological characters (including rules of connectivity) and the same biochemical (and immunological) properties. At least in principle, the category could be defined by a common repertoire of "open" genes (able to be transcribed and translated into proteins), in other words, by the *differentiated state* of the cells.

On the other hand, microphysiological recordings of single cells within a category disclose clear-cut differences. For instance, in the area of projection of eye muscles on the cerebellar vermis, a given Purkinje cell will respond by a *decreased* firing rate when the right lateral rectus muscle is stretched, yet another one will respond by an increased firing rate when the right median rectus muscle now is stretched (Schwarz & Tomlinson, 1977). In some areas of the cerebellum, Purkinje cells will be characterized by several sensory modalities, in other areas by single ones. Therefore, within a given cell category, a remarkable functional diversity exists. The word *singularity* (Changeux, 1980) can be proposed to qualify this diversity. In principle, the singularity of any cell within a given category can be described by the repertoire of its afferent and efferent synapses, in other words by its precise connectivity. At this level of resolution, little true redundancy exists within a cell category.

Comparative anatomy of the nervous system of vertebrates and invertebrates discloses two different evolutionary trends. Starting from a diffuse (coelenterates), highly redundant, metamerized (worms) organization, one trend is to increase the number of categories without changing the number of cells; the number of categories therefore approximates the number of cells. This is the case of the nervous system of Aplysia (Kandel, 1976) and Nematodes (Sulston & Horvitz, 1977). Another trend, which manifested itself at least twice in the course of evolution, in Cephalopodes (Young, 1971) and in Vertebrates, results in an increase of the number of cells within a category rather than in the number of categories. A diversification by "singularization" then takes place. Interestingly, this diversification often conserves some common functional features or discloses some regularity in the distribution of properties among cells from a given area that may thus form a *map* (of a sensory or motor organ or of another nerve center). The first evolutive trend could be referred to as "evolution by categorization," the second as "evolution by singularization." The complexity of the first group of nervous systems would be directly linked to the repertoire of active genes in any given cell, but this would not be necessarily the case in the second one.

THE ONTOGENESIS OF THE COMPLEXITY OF THE NERVOUS SYSTEM

The differentiation of the neural ectoderm and of the different cell categories, the morphogenesis of the ganglia and/or neural tube are processes of embryonic development that might follow rules similar to those of any other organ of the body. They are thus excluded from this discussion, which is limited to the complexity linked to connectivity.

Complexity of the Genome and Complexity of the Nervous System Compared

A rather crude and naive manner to relate the organization of the genome with that of the nervous system is to compare the weight of DNA in the fertilized egg and the total number of cells in the adult nervous system. *Drosophila* diploid genome consists of $.24 \times 10^{-6}$ µg DNA and there are about 100,000 neurons. In the mouse, the fertilized egg contains 27 times more DNA than in *Drosophila* but the nerve cells are, at least, 60 times more abundant. Man possesses 2 billion to 16.5 billion nerve cells and nearly the same amount of DNA as the mouse per diploid genome. Hybridization experiments between total DNA of chimpanzee and man reveal not more than a 1.1% difference of nucleotide sequences (King & Wilson, 1975). Finally, the estimation of the *absolute* number of different structural genes (of average size) gives astonishingly small numbers of 5000 to 6000 in *Drosophila* and

20,000 to 100,000 in mammals. In addition, only a fraction of them is expected to be unique to the nervous system. The complex organization of the
nervous system thus develops during the course of evolution, starting from a
small set of genes. Moreover, at least in vertebrates and particularly in mammals, a remarkable *nonlinear* relationship is noticed between the evolution of
the complexity of the genome and that of the fine anatomy of the nervous
system.

A formal solution to this paradox is that inasmuch as *no simple* relationship exists between gene and neuronal morphology, *combinations* of genes
might be used to label each cell and each synapse of a given cell (see Monod,
1980). The number of genes would be, in any instance, sufficient to create a
large repertoire of labels. However, this reasoning does not explicitly deal
with the *nonlinearity* mentioned in the preceding paragraph.

Another plausible solution is that a *combinatory* mechanism of another
nature accounts for the diversification of nerve cells and requires only a small
number of genes.

Limits of the Genetic Determinism

Evidence for such a combinatory mechanism might come from the analysis
of the limits occurring in the genetic determinism of the functional organization of the nervous system. It is difficult to define the minimal effect of a gene
mutation because it is a priori determined by the sensitivity of the method of
mutant selection. For example, some known lesions, caused by point mutations, affect: (1) Purkinje cells (PCD) or granular cells in the mouse (weaver)
(Caviness & Rakic, 1978; Sotelo & Privat, 1978); or (2) a given photo receptor
cell (e.g., R7) common to all the ommatidia of *Drosophila* eyes (Harris,
Stark, & Walker, 1976); and (3) probably one class of synapses between parallel fibers and Purkinje cell dendrites in the *staggerer* mouse (Landis &
Sidman, 1978; Mariani & Changeux, 1980a). The minimal known effect of
gene mutations seems to affect all cells that belong to a given *category*.

Limits in the genetic determinism are also expressed by the phenotypic variance of the fine neuroanatomy of isogenic animals (Levinthal, Macagno, &
Levinthal, 1976). This variance is significant in small invertebrates like
Daphnia (Macagno, Lopresti, & Levinthal, 1973) where it affects the number
of morphological synapses within a given category, it may be more important, though difficult to estimate, in mammals where the number of neurons
is large (Wimer, Wimer, Vaughn, Barber, Balvanz, & Chernow, 1976).

The existence of such limits justifies the concept of a "genetic envelope"
that contains the invariant characters of the adult nervous system but also allows significant phenotypic variance.

Transient Structural Redundancy: An Ontogenetic Mechanism of Amplification with a Low Gene Cost

The setting out of neuronal *somas* in highly "categorized" nervous systems such as that of *Caenorhabditis elegans* (and presumably all the nervous systems with a fixed number of cells) takes place through a sequence of cell divisions and differentiation (including cell death) that follow invariant patterns.

This is not the case in the nervous systems of high vertebrates. For instance, the lineage of Purkinje cells in the cerebellum of allophenic mice (Mullen, 1978) does not suggest any simple relationship between the adult distribution of these cells and the pattern of division of their immature precursors. After their last division, the precursors of the Purkinje cells migrate to their final location in a quasi-random manner. When they reach the cerebellar cortex they likely are all equivalent. A similar situation may occur during the development of the cerebral cortex.

A similar redundancy has been noticed later in development when functional synapses become established. For instance, in the newborn rat, up to five climbing fibers make functional contacts with each Purkinje cell (Crepel, Delhaye-Bouchaud, & Mariani, 1976; Mariani & Changeux, 1980a,b, 1981), but, in the adult, only a single one persists (Eccles, Llinas, & Sasaki, 1966). A similar situation has been reported in the case of sympathetic and parasympathetic (Lichtman, 1977; Lichtman & Purves, 1980) ganglia and in the well-known case of the motor end plate (Redfern, 1970, reviewed in Changeux, 1979). It may simply result from the fact that the elements of structure that determine the formation of the early contacts are not unique to each individual contact but common to the *category* of contacts (for instance the climbing fiber–Purkinje cell synapses). Again, the setting out of this redundant synaptic organization does not require a large number of genes.

A common feature of this redundancy is its *transient* character. During development, significant cell death (up to 40%) occurs and, at later stages, many of the synaptic contacts regress (Cowan, 1979) (up to 80%). These regressive phenomena accompany the "singularization" of the nerve cells.

The Activity of the Developing Neuronal Network: Its Contribution to Epigenesis

Classical cybernetics considers nerve activity mainly as an intermediate component of the input–output relationship of the adult organism in its environment. Here, the activity of the developing neuronal network is viewed as an *internal* signaling mechanism that plays a morphogenetic role during embryogenesis and postnatal development. The word activity will describe any process that directly or indirectly results in a change of electrical properties of the neuronal membrane, including the propagation of action potentials, electrical coupling, chemical transmission and modulation, and, eventually, the evoked release of so-called "trophic" factors.

Various electrical phenomena have been recorded during early stages of development, even in the egg. For instance, *Xenopus* oocytes respond to acetylcholine by a depolarization and to dopamine or serotonin by a hyperpolarization (Kusano, Miledi, & Stinnakre, 1977). In *Amblyostoma,* at the early stages of neural tube formation a difference of membrane potential appears between the ectodermic (about 30 mV) and embryonic neural cells (-44 mV) (Warner, 1973). At later stages regenerative phenomena develop only in this last class of cells.

Spontaneous movements are observed in chick embryos as early as 3–5 days in ovo. These movements last throughout embryogenesis and are neurogenic of origin (Hamburger, 1970). Even growth cones may release significant amounts of neurotransmitter (Cohen, 1980). Such spontaneous neural activity has been recorded in embryos of all groups of vertebrates including man (Bergstrøm, 1969). Most often the spontaneous firing of the neurons occurs as bursts of action potentials. Similar oscillatory behavior of membrane properties has been recorded in many different categories of cells (*Aplysia* neurons, Purkinje fibers of the heart, pancreatic islets (Berridge & Rapp, 1979)). In all instances the ionic mechanism for generation of these oscillations appears rather simple: two "rapid" Na^+ and K^+ ionic channels for the action potential and two "slow" K^+ and Ca^{++} channels for the pacemaker. Genesis of spontaneous activity probably requires only a few structural genes and, in addition, the same gene products can be utilized in different cells and organs.

Sense organs also generate spontaneous activity even before they begin to respond to physical stimuli from the outside world. This is the case for retina ganglion cells (Cavaggioni, 1968) and for vestibular receptors (Wilson & Melvill-Jones, 1979). In a general manner, embryonic sensory receptors may behave as *peripheral* oscillators that contribute to the spontaneous activity recorded in the centers.

Of course, as soon as the sense organs become functional, the contribution of the evoked activity circulating in the developing nervous system becomes more and more significant. It is worth noting that the nervous systems where the most striking nonlinearity exists between genomic versus neural complexity are precisely those where the period of postnatal synaptogenesis lasts longer. This is, of course, highly suggestive of a plausible role of evoked activity, in addition to the spontaneous one, in the regulation of synapse formation.

The working hypothesis that spontaneous and evoked activity plays a morphogenetic role during development of the nervous system offers a significant number of possibilities. The activity propagated in the developing network is a long-distance mechanism of interaction between cells and even organs. The "convergence" and "divergence" properties of neurons make possible the integration of many signals at the neuronal level. A *combinatory mechanism* can thus be generated by the propagated activity.

THE SELECTIVE STABILIZATION OF DEVELOPING SYNAPSES: A PLAUSIBLE MECHANISM FOR THE SINGULARIZATION OF NERVE CELLS

The theory of epigenesis by selective stabilization (Changeux, 1972; Changeux, Courrège, & Danchin, 1973; Changeux, Courrège, Danchin, & Lasry, 1981; Changeux & Danchin, 1974, 1976) deals with the main issues presented in the previous section. The mechanism proposed is a combinatory mechanism able to generate a considerable diversification of nerve cells on the basis of a small number of genetic determinants. It primarily concerns the highly singularized nervous system of vertebrates (particularly mammals and primates).

The stage of development that was referred to as structural redundancy is taken as the initial state. The theory was originally designed for developing synapses but can be extended to the neuronal somas. At this stage, excitatory (or inhibitory) synapses of the considered category may exist under at least three states, labile (L), stable (S), and degenerate (D). Only the L and S states transmit nerve impulses and the acceptable transitions between states are $L \rightarrow S$, $L \rightarrow D$, and $S \rightarrow L$. The evolution of the connective state of a given synapse σ is governed by the total message of activity, $U(t)$, afferent to the postsynaptic soma during a prior time interval. This regulatory function of the neuronal soma is referred to as its "evolutive power" Δ. The maximal connectivity, at the peak of transient redundancy, the main stages of development of the network of synaptic connections, the evolutive power of the soma and its integrative properties Φ, in other words the rules of growth and stabilization by activity of the redundant and labile synaptic contacts, is a determinate expression of the genetic program (the genetic "envelope" of the network).

Neuronal graphs ($C\Sigma$) provide a model of the connective organization of the network where the synapses are labeled by the elements of Σ. If Θ and η respectively represent the rules of propagation and "memorization" by the soma of the afferent multimessages, then one may consider a mathematical structure

$$R = (C, \Sigma, \Theta, n, \Phi, \Delta) \text{ or "neuronal program."}$$

The "actualization" of R for a given afferent multimessage during the "critical period" of synaptic plasticity results in the stabilization of a particular set of synapses from the graph ($C\Sigma$) while the other ones regress.

A first consequence of the theory offers a plausible mechanism for the recording of a temporal sequence of nerve impulses as a stable trace that can be described in terms of network growth (and not solely in terms of synapse efficacy (see Kandel, 1976)). This trace is printed as a particular pattern of connective organization that exists *before* the critical period of stabilization. It differs from instructive mechanisms that assume, for instance, that a particular message directs the growth of nerve endings towards suitable targets or causes the appearance of new molecular species. The proposed mechanism is a strictly *selective* one.

A second consequence, which can be demonstrated rigorously, is that the same afferent multimessage may stabilize different connective organizations that nevertheless result in the same input–output relationships. What we referred to as "variability" (Changeux et al., 1973) may account for the phenotypic variance noticed in isogenic individuals. It, of course, accounts for the *singularization* of nerve cells within a given *category* at the stage of transient synaptic redundancy. According to these views several different connective combinations may result in the *same* behavior. The code for behavior would thus be "degenerate."

Finally, the genes that compose the genetic envelope, in particular those that determine the rules of growth and stabilization of synaptic contacts, might be "open," in the highly singularized nervous systems, in all the nerve cells that belong to the *same category*. Thus the cost in genes might be rather low. The development of an amplification device by transient structural redundancy associated with a combinatory epigenetic mechanism accounts for the paradoxical nonlinearity noticed between the complexity of the genome and that of the connective organization of mammalian nervous systems.

EXPERIMENTAL TEST OF THE THEORY

Only fragmentary data are yet available. The central issue of the theory (that synapse stabilization and elimination is the mechanism for nerve cell singularization and thus for the development of their specific functional modalities) still requires an unambiguous demonstration. The experimental observations reported here concern only two systems: (1) the neuromuscular junction from chick embryo and newborn rat; and (2) the cerebellar cortex from rat and mouse. Moreover, only *data from our laboratory are reviewed*.

Consequences of the Chronic Paralysis of Chick Embryos on the Development of the Neuromuscular Junction

When nicotinic antagonists such as curare, flaxedil, or snake α-toxins are chronically injected into yolk sacs of chick embryos, spontaneous movements of the embryos are blocked without systematically causing their death. (In adults, death results from the paralysis of the respiratory muscles.) This essentially postsynaptic (the antagonists bind to the acetylcholine receptor) and peripheral (the pharmacological agents do not cross the blood brain barrier) blocking has consequences both on the pre- and postsynaptic sides of the motor endplates.

A significant decrease of the total content of the *presynaptic* enzyme choline acetyltransferase (responsible for acetylcholine synthesis) in the muscle and sciatic nerve takes place after paralysis by α-bungarotoxin from the third to twelfth day of incubation (Betz, Bourgeois, & Changeux, 1980; Giacobini, Filogamo, Weber, Boquet, & Changeux, 1973; Giacobini, Robecchi, Giacobini, Filogamo, & Changeux, 1975). The total number of motor neurons that persist in the spinal cord also decreases below the normal level under the same conditions. However, different conditions of paralysis (such as by curare instead of α-bungarotoxin from the sixth to ninth day in ovo) has the opposite effect (Pittman & Oppenheim, 1979). Many more motor neurons persist in the paralyzed compared to control embryos. Under these conditions, paralysis prevents cell death. In any case, and in agreement with the selective stabilization hypothesis, cell death, and therefore the survival of the adult neurons, is regulated by the activity of the neuromuscular junction.

At the *postsynaptic* level, chronic paralysis does not interfere with the subsynaptic accumulation of the acetylcholine receptor but interferes with the disappearance of the extrajunctional receptor (Betz et al., 1980). More extrasynaptic receptors persist in the paralyzed embryo. Because the half-life of the receptor molecule does not change under these conditions, the regulation must take place at the level of the receptor protein synthetic machinery. In the course of normal development, the neurally evoked electrical activity of the muscle thus represses the synthesis of acetylcholine receptor. An involvement of Ca^{++} and/or cyclic nucleotides as "second messengers" in this regulation appears plausible (Betz & Changeux, 1979).

Chronic postsynaptic block prevents the localization of the degradative enzyme acetylcholinesterase. Activity of the muscle is *required* for the local accumulation of the enzyme in the basal lamina that covers the subsynaptic membrane (Giacobini et al., 1973; Gordon, Perry, Tuffery, & Vrbova, 1974; Oppenheim, Pittman, Gray, & Madredrut, 1978; Rubin, Schuetze, Weill, &

Fischbach, 1980). Because the transmission efficiency of the endplate depends on the synaptic content of acetylcholinesterase, this regulation can be taken as a model for the effect of "disuse" or "experience" on the functional (and biochemical) properties of a synapse.

Effect of Chronic Stimulation of Chick Embryo Spinal Cord on the Pattern of Motor Endplates

In the chick, the wing muscles, *latissimus dorsi*, receive two distinct types of innervation. The slow *anterior* muscle (ALD) shows several endplates distributed at approximately equal distances along the muscle fiber, whereas the fast *posterior* muscle (PLD) receives a single focal endplate in the middle of the fiber.

Cross-innervation experiments in the embryo have shown that the nerve, not the muscle, determines the pattern of endplates (Hnik, Jirmanova, Vyklicky, & Zelena, 1967; Zelena & Jirmanova, 1979). Moreover, during development, the programs of neurally evoked spontaneous activity differ in the two muscles: In 15-day-old embryos, the ALD shows a sustained low activity of around .2–1 Hz, whereas the PLD shows high frequency bursts of activity around 8 Hz interrupted by periods of silence (Gordon, Purves, & Vrbova, 1977).

To test the hypothesis that the activity of the nerve regulates or even determines the pattern of endplates, electrodes were chronically implanted around the brachial spinal cord in 7-day embryos in ovo by the method developed by Renaud, Le Douarin, and Khaskiye (1978) and electric pulses delivered at .5 Hz frequency from the 10th–15th day of incubation. Quantitative analysis of the number and distribution of clusters of acetylcholine receptor (Toutant, Bourgeois, Toutant, Renaud, Le Douarin, & Changeux, 1980) and of patches of acetylcholinesterase activity (Toutant, 1981) discloses a significant increase of their number per individual PLD muscle fiber and per total PLD muscle (by a factor of 1.8 to 2.0). However, the distribution of the multiple clusters of acetylcholine receptor that appear in the normally focally innervated PLD is not as regular as in ALD. The parallel evolution of the clusters of acetylcholine receptor and esterase supports the conclusion that the chronic stimulation of the PLD muscle with a program close to that of ALD resulted in a distributed pattern of endplates over the fiber. An electrophysiological demonstration of this point, however, is missing.

A still theoretical, and thus speculative, biochemical mechanism (Changeux et al., 1981) has been proposed to account for the epigenetic dependence of the ALD and PLD synaptic topologies on the afferent multimessage resulting from the spontaneous activity of the spinal cord during development. In its initial state the muscle fiber receives exploratory motor nerve endings (originating from the same neuron) at multiple points randomly distributed along the fiber. At each of these points the nerve endings release acetylcholine and, as a consequence, the neurally evoked activity of the muscle fiber stops the synthesis of receptor. The biochemical postulates of the model are restricted to: (1) the interconversion of the receptor protein from a labile L form to an A form, which may aggregate under a nerve terminal (whereas the L does not) but still diffuses laterally in the muscle membrane; (2) the release by the nerve endings of an "anterograde factor" with a finite half-life, the amount of factor liberated being directly linked to the afferent multimessage $U(t)$; once liberated, the factor triggers the transformation of L to A; (3) the aggregation of the receptor begins and continues with a faster rate when the local concentration of A reaches a threshold value. The computer simulation of the mathematical model confirms that the biochemical hypotheses made are sufficient to obtain a distributed pattern of acetylcholine receptor clusters (nevertheless in numbers smaller than the initial number of contacts) when the afferent multimessage is continuous and a focal pattern when it is in bursts. Even though plausible, none of the biochemical hypotheses made have been demonstrated experimentally.

Experimental Analysis of the Regression of Polyneuronal Innervation of Skeletal Muscle in Newborn Rats

At birth, in the rat, acetylcholine receptor and esterase are localized at the motor endplate, which receives several functional nerve terminals originating from different motor neurons. Twenty days after birth, a single nerve ending persists per endplate. This regression coincides with the segregation of the motor units. In the simplest situation, each motor neuron innervates the same number of muscle fibers (motor unit) but no regularity exists in the relative distribution of the muscle fibers in any given motor unit. In other words, the muscle fibers from different motor units are randomly mixed (review in Brown, Jansen, & Van Essen, 1976). In a first attempt to demonstrate an effect of activity on the regression of multiple innervation, the tendon of the sartorius muscle was sectioned in newborn rats. As a consequence, the mechanical activity of the muscle becomes negligible and an important delay in the regression of the multiinnervation takes place (Benoit & Changeux, 1975). The paralysis of the motor nerve by a cuff of local anesthetic has the same effect (Benoit & Changeux, 1978). Finally, chronic electrical stimulation accelerates the regression of the multiple innervation. In conclusion, the stabilization of one motor nerve ending per muscle fiber is an "active" process that nerve activity regulates.

A theoretical model (Gouzé et al., 1983) accounts for this evolution, if one assumes that: (1) a *retrograde* postsynaptic factor, produced in limiting amounts by the muscle fibers, is required for the stabilization of the motor nerve ending; (2) an uptake of the retrograde factor takes place when an impulse reaches the nerve terminal; and (3) an *internal* presynaptic factor, which circulates inside the neuron and its axonal branches, is present in limiting amounts and combines with the retrograde factor to yield an active complex that triggers the stabilization of the nerve ending.

Postnatal Evolution of the Olivo–Cerebellar Relationships in Rat and Mouse

If the occurrence of transient polyneuronal innervation were unique to the neuromuscular junction, this phenomenon could not be taken as a model for a general mechanism of neurogenesis. It was thus essential to examine, in this respect, another system. The innervation of the Purkinje cells from cerebellar cortex by the climbing fibers (which originate from olivary neurons) appears adequate because, in the adult, only one climbing fiber innervates each Purkinje cell. Interestingly, in newborn rats, *several* functional climbing fibers (up to five) end on each Purkinje cell (Crépel et al., 1976) but all of them, except one, are eliminated later during development (Mariani & Changeux, 1980b, 1981). An important spontaneous activity is recorded in the system (Mariani & Changeux, 1981) but its contribution to the stabilization of the adult synapses is not demonstrated. On the other hand, the elimination of granular cells in the newborn by X-ray irradiation or mutation is followed by the maintenance, in the adult, of the multiinnervation of the Purkinje cell by several climbing fibers (Crépel & Mariani, 1976; Mariani & Changeux, 1980a,b; Mariani, Crépel, Mikoshiba, Changeux, & Sotelo, 1977).

CONCLUSION

The selective stabilization as a theory of developing synapses brings one, albeit necessarily limited answer to the questions raised by the ontogenesis of neuron complexity at a low gene cost. It offers a plausible mechanism for nerve cell diversification based on the combination of elementary activities working on a redundant and labile framework of developing synapses.

This mechanism is still hypothetical but can be experimentally tested and thus might be useful. Research presently develops in our laboratory along two lines: (1) the identification at the *molecular level* of the mechanism responsible for the stabilization of developing synapses such as the interaction of the acetylcholine receptor with the basal lamina (Labat-Robert, Saitoh,

Godeau, Robert, & Changeux, 1980) or with internal periplasmic or cytoskeletal proteins (Cartaud, Sobel, Rousselet, Devaux, & Changeux, 1981; Rousselet, Cartaud, & Devaux, 1979; Saitoh, Wennogle, & Changeux, 1979); the covalent modifications of the receptor protein during development (Saitoh & Changeux, 1981); the isolation of retrograde factors (Henderson, Huchet, & Changeux, 1981); and the role of activity on these various processes; (2) the understanding of the role played by this mechanism of synapse stabilization and elimination in the differentiation of complex networks. Its extension to more elaborate systems, such as the visual cortex, appears worth trying. Finally, theoretical work still has to be done to relate the selective stabilization of synapses and the development of maps.

ACKNOWLEDGMENTS

We thank B. Holton for her criticisms of the manuscript, T. Sciuto and E. Couelle for typing it. This work was supported by grants from the Muscular Dystrophy Association of America, the Fondation Fyssen, the Fondation de France, the Fondation pour la Recherche Médicale, the Collège de France, the Délégation Générale à la Recherche Scientifique et Technique, the Centre National de la Recherche Scientifique, the Institut National de la Santé et de la Recherche Médicale and the Commissariat à l'Energie Atomique.

REFERENCES

Benoit, P., & Changeux, J. P. (1975). *Brain Research, 99,* 354–358.
Benoit, P., & Changeux, J. P. (1978). *Brain Research, 149,* 89–96.
Bergstrom, R. (1969). In *Brain and early behavior.* R. J. Robinson (ed.), pp. 15–42. New York, Academic Press.
Berridge, M. J., & Rapp, P. E. (1979). *J. Exp. Biol., 81,* 217–279.
Betz, H., & Changeux, J. P. (1979). *Nature, 278,* 749–752.
Betz, H., Bourgeois, J. P., & Changeux, J. P. (1980). *J. Physiol., 302,* 197–218.
Brown, M. C., Jansen, J. K. S., & Van Essen, D. (1976). *J. Physiol., (Lond.), 261,* 387–422.
Cartaud, J., Sobel, A., Rousselet, A., Devaux, P. F., & Changeux, J. P. (1981). *J. Cell. Biol., 90,* 418–426.
Cavaggioni, A. (1968). *Pfüger's Arch., 304,* 75–80.
Caviness, V., & Rakiĉ, P. (1978). *Ann. Rev. Neurosci., 1,* 297–326.
Changeux, J. P. (1972). *Communications, 18,* 37–47.
Changeux, J. P., Courrège, Ph., & Danchin, A. (1973). *Proc. Natl. Acad. Sci. USA, 70,* 2974–2978.
Changeux, J. P., & Danchin, A. (1974). In *L'unité de l'homme.* E. Morin & M. Piatteli (eds.), pp. 320–357. Paris, Le Seuil.
Changeux, J. P., & Danchin, A. (1976). *Nature, 264,* 705–712.
Changeux, J. P. (1979). In *The Neurosciences, fourth study program.* The MIT Press, Cambridge & London, pp. 749–778.
Changeux, J. P. (1980). *Annuaire du Collège de France, 80,* 309–343.

Changeux, J. P., Courrège, Ph., Danchin, A., & Lasry, J. M. (1981). *C. R. Acad. Sci. Paris, 292*, 449–453.

Cohen, S. A. (1980). *Proc. Natl. Acad. Sci. USA, 77*, 644–648.

Cowan, W. M. (1979). In *The Neurosciences, fourth study program*. F. O. Schmitt & F. G. Worden (eds.). The MIT Press, Cambridge, MA. pp. 59–81.

Crepel, F., Delhaye-Bouchard, N., & Mariani, J. (1976). *J. Neurobiol., 7*, 579–582.

Eccles, J. C., Llinas, R., & Sasaki, K. (1966). *J. Physiol. (Lond.), 182*, 268–296.

Giacobini, G., Filogamo, G., Weber, M., Boquet, P., & Changeux, J. P. (1973). *Proc. Natl. Acad. Sci. USA, 70*, 1708–1712.

Giacobini-Robecchi, M. G., Giacobini, G., Filogamo, G., & Changeux, J. P. (1975). *Brain Res., 83*, 107–121.

Gordon, T., Perry, R., Tuffery, A. R., & Vrbova, G. (1974). *Cell Tissue Res., 115*, 13–25.

Gordon, T., Purves, R., & Vrbova, G. (1977). *J. Physiol. (Lond.), 269*, 535–547.

Gouzé, J. L., Lasry, J. M., & Changeux, J. P. (1983). *Biol. Cybern., 46*, 207–215.

Hamburger, V. (1970). In *The Neurosciences, second study program*. F. O. Schmitt (ed.). The Rockefeller University Press, New York, pp. 141–151.

Harris, W. A., Stark, W. S., & Walker, J. A. (1976). *J. Physiol., 256*, 415–439.

Henderson, C. E., Huchet, M., & Changeux, J. P. (1981). *Proc. Natl. Acad. Sci., 78,*(4), 2625–2629.

Hnik, P., Jirmanova, I., Vyklicky, L., & Zelena, J. (1967). *J. Physiol. (Lond.), 193*, 309–325.

Kandel, E. (1976). In *Cellular basis of behavior*. W.H. Freeman, San Francisco.

King, M. C., & Wilson, A. C. (1975). *Science, 188*, 107–116.

Kusano, K., Miledi, R., & Stinnakre, J. (1977). *Nature, 270*, 739–741.

Labat-Robert, J., Saitoh, T., Godeau, G., Robert, L., & Changeux, J. P. (1980). *FEBS Lett., 120*, 259–263.

Landis, D. M., & Sidman, R. L. (1978). *J. Comp. Neurol., 179*, 831–863.

Levinthal, F., Macagno, E., & Levinthal, C. (1976). *Cold Spring Harbor Symp. Quant. Biol., 40*, 321–332.

Lichtman, J. W. (1977). *J. Physiol. (Lond.), 273*, 155–177.

Lichtman, J. W., & Purves, D. (1980). *J. Physiol. (Lond.), 301*, 213–228.

Macagno, E., Lopresti, V., & Levinthal, C. (1973). *Proc. Natl. Acad. Sci. USA, 70*, 57–61.

Mariani, J., Crépel, F., Mikoshiba, K., Changeux, J. P., & Sotelo, C. (1977). *Phil. Trans. Roy. Soc. B., 281*, 1–28.

Mariani, J., & Changeux, J. P. (1980a). *J. Neurobiol., 11*, 41–50.

Mariani, J., & Changeux, J. P. (1980b). *C.R. Acad. Sci. Paris, 291*, 97–100.

Mariani, J., & Changeux, J. P. (1981). *J. Neurosci., 1*, 696–709.

Monod, J. (1980). In *Language and Learning*. M. Piatelli-Palmarini (ed.). Harvard University Press, Cambridge.

Mullen, R. J. (1978). In *The clonal basis of development*. S. Subtelny & I. M. Sussex (eds.) Academic Press, New York.

Oppenheim, R. W., Pittman, R., Gray, M., & Madredrut, J. L. (1978). *J. Comp. Neurol., 179*, 619–640.

Palay, S., & Chan-Palay, V. (1974). *Cerebellar cortex*. Springer-Verlag, Berlin.

Pittman, R., & Oppenheim, R. W. (1979). *J. Comp. Neurol., 187*, 425–446.

Renaud, D., Le Douarin, G., & Khaskiye, A. (1978). *Exp. Neurol., 60*, 189–200.

Rousselet, A., Cartaud, J., & Devaux, P. F. (1979). *C.R. Acad. Sci. Paris. D, 289*, 461–463.

Rubin, L. L., Schuetze, S. M., Weill, C. L., & Fischbach, G. D. (1980). *Nature, 283*, 264–267.

Saitoh, T., Wennogle, L., & Changeux, J. P. (1979). *FEBS Lett., 108*, 489–494.

Saitoh, T., & Changeux, J. P. (1981). *Proc. Natl. Acad. Sci. USA, 78*, 4430–4434.

Schwarz, D. W., & Tomlinson, R. D. (1977). *Exp. Brain Res., 27*, 101–111.

Sotelo, C., & Privat, A. (1978). *Acta Neuropathol. (Berl.), 43*, 19–34.

Sulston, J. E., & Horvitz, H. R. (1977). *Develop. Biol., 56*, 110–246.

Toutant, M., Bourgeois, J. P., Toutant, J. P., Renaud, D., Le Douarin, G., & Changeux, J. P. (1980). *Develop. Biol., 76,* 384–395.

Toutant, M., Toutant, J. P., Renaud, D., Le Douarin, G., & Changeux, J. P. (1981). *C.R. Acad. Sci. Paris, III, 292,* 771–775.

Warner, A. E. (1973). *J. Physiol., 235,* 267–286.

Wilson, V. J., & Melvill-Jones, G. (1979). *Mammalian vestibular physiology.* Plenum Press, New York and London.

Wimer, R. E., Wimer, C. C., Vaughn, J. E., Barber, R. P., Balvanz, B. A., & Chernow, C. R. (1976). *Brain Res., 118,* 219–243.

Young, J. Z. (1971). *The anatomy of the nervous system of Octopus vulgaris.* Oxford, Clarendon Press.

Zelena, J., & Jirmanova, I. (1979). *Exp. Neurol., 38,* 272–285.

6 The Rules of Elemental Synaptic Plasticity

William B. Levy
Nancy L. Desmond
Department of Neurological Surgery
University of Virginia School of Medicine

The hypothesis that learning and memory involve neuronal modifications antedates the advent of the synaptic doctrine. In 1862, Herbert Spencer postulated that memory storage occurred via altering one cell's ability to excite another cell as a function of prior activity. According to Ramon y Cajal (1911), Tanzi proposed that neural networks develop their functional capacities by altering synaptic interactions. Some time later, and benefiting from few, if any, relevant experimental facts, Hebb (1949) correctly predicted the apparent essence of the elemental, synaptic learning rule that forms the cellular basis of perceptual development and associative learning and memory.

In formulating elemental learning rules, Hebb and succeeding theoreticians posit rules that, when incorporated into a suitable neuroanatomical model, yield systems with capabilities analogous to some mammalian cognitive functions (e.g. associative memory, concept formation, and pattern recognition). This performance and any inherent mathematical elegance of the system are the primary arguments for the biological reality of the proposed synaptic process. Because many of these theories are largely unfettered by biological fact (in the Hebbian tradition), a rich array of synaptic learning rules are proposed, of which only a small number are likely to resemble actual synaptic physiology.

This chapter proposes rules similar to some postulated from purely theoretical considerations. However, the rules are presented here in a context strongly limited by recent experiments on adult neural plasticity. Influencing these hypotheses are the rationale used by Hebb and other theoreticians and two additional, interacting reasons:

1. The elemental rules are useful building blocks for cognitive function.
2. The rules are mutually complementary.
3. The cellular changes are not unreasonable given our current knowledge of cell biology.

Rather than focusing exclusively upon the first rationale with a detailed mathematical exposition of its implications, this chapter emphasizes the second and third rationales, which ensure that the elemental rules are coherent and biologically feasible.

In subsequent sections, the regulatory principles are listed for excitatory synapses followed by a teleological discussion of the utility and parsimony of these rules, their mathematical expression, and some biological data justifying the results. Following the discussion of excitatory synaptic modification rules are similar sections concerning inhibitory synapses.

EXCITATORY SYNAPSES

The Postulated Rules

Four rules are postulated to govern changes in connectivity and synaptic efficacy at excitatory synapses within the mature brain.

1a. Convergent coactivity increases synaptic efficacy at active synapses (the Hebb rule).
1b. Presynaptic inactivity during postsynaptic activity decreases synaptic efficacy at the inactive synapse (anti-Hebb rule).
2. The receptivity of (or posssibly the request by) a postsynaptic target for new innervation varies as an inverse function of its activity (postsynaptic growth rule).
3. An afferent's propensity for axonal growth and competitiveness for claiming an available postsynaptic site is dynamically regulated, increasing with heightened levels of activity and decreasing with lowered levels of activity (axonal growth rule).

Partial Explication and Teleology

The overriding theoretical position directing the selection of "useful" rules is that individual synapses would be extremely useful memory units. Such a unit would store information that can help predict the activity of converging afferents and the postsynaptic cell. This synaptic function is not original. Many theoreticians (e.g. Amari, 1977; Anderson, 1968; Kohonen, 1970; Marr, 1971; Uttley, 1976a, 1976b, 1976c) propose this idea because it explains various aspects of associative memory and also forms the basis of higher functions such as concept formation. Thus, the elemental rules that help synapses store the appropriate correlations and that contribute to the ability of cells to form concepts and perform pattern recognition are generally consistent with current directions in neurodynamics.

Excitatory Rule 1a: Hebb Rule.   Thirty years ago, Hebb (1949) proposed that associative learning and memory emerge from microscopic associations occurring at the level of cell-to-cell synaptic interactions. As a general scheme, the operative principles governing these microscopic associations are well known and almost universally accepted by neural modelers. The Hebb rule states that when a presynaptic afferent is coactive with a postsynaptic cell, the synaptic efficacy between the two elements increases. With recurring associated activity, the efficacy of each synapse resembles the correlation between the activity of the presynaptic afferent and the postsynaptic cell. This rule is useful in various neuropsychological processes, including concept formation (Anderson, 1979), associative recall (Kohonen, 1977), and visual development (Cooper, Liberman, & Oja, 1979).

The three remaining excitatory rules are formalized to optimize synaptic participation in concept formation and prediction and to fit the experimental data.

Excitatory Rule 1b: Anti-Hebb Rule—Depression[1].   Ranck (1964), Rosenblatt (1967), and most exactly Stent (1973) propose a complementary microscopic law of dissociation. Specifically, decreases in synaptic efficacy occur when the postsynaptic cell is active concurrently with presynaptic inactivity. Kohonen, Lehtio, and Rovano (1974) and Cooper et al. (1979) incorporate a similar assumption in their elemental learning rules. This anti-Hebb rule allows for a self-organizing system by permitting the removal of inappropriate correlations. In the same vein, this rule allows for unlearning when an individual feature of a temporally discrete concept is no longer associated with the original concept because of the dissociation of two events.

A second anti-Hebb rule, which our experimental impressions do not support, should be distinguished. This other anti-Hebb rule preducts depression when the presynaptic element is active and the postsynaptic cell is inactive. Cooper et al. (1979) incorporate this rule in their elemental learning rules. Although we agree that the nervous system ought to appreciate this type of noncorrelation, we prefer to include this learning rule at inhibitory synapses (*vide infra*).

Together, rules 1a and 1b provide a self-organizational capability whereby a system with initially random connections forms "specific" (i.e., properly

---

[1]The term *depression* is equivalent to *depotentiation* as discussed by Levy (Chapter 1, this volume).

specified) connections based on correlated activity. As a result, the postsynaptic cell comes to identify concepts (specific groupings of afferent activity) via potentiation. Simultaneously, the activity of synapses is depressed if their existence indicates inappropriate correlations relative to the history of afferent activity. Finally, these two rules also provide a developmental mechanism for the formation of topographic mappings in sensory systems where correlated activity of nearby receptors ensures mapping specificity (cf. Singer, chapter 2, this volume).

Excitatory Rule 2: Postsynaptic Growth.   Rule 2 states that postsynaptic *in*activity produces a postsynaptic condition compatible with new excitatory innervation (and vice versa for postsynaptic hyperactivity). This dynamic rule controls the maximum number of synapses a cell can receive, with the maximum a function of the time-averaged activity of the postsynaptic cell. Thus, the maximum number of synapses permitted increases as the overall postsynaptic excitation decreases.

Three hypoactive conditions lead to receptivity (or even request by) a postsynaptic neuron for innervation: (1) gross inactivity of its afferents; (2) uncorrelated (i.e., asynchronous) afferent activity, with depression consistently removing potentiation; and (3) correlated afferent activity whose postsynaptic expression (cell firing or large amounts of localized dendritic excitation) is blocked by simultaneous, convergent inhibition.

Excitatory Rule 3: Axonal Growth.   Rule 3 is the presynaptic complement of Rule 2 and defines afferents with the potential for synaptogenesis. Synaptogenesis is theorized to be limited by the dynamically regulated amount of functional presynaptic surface area. This presynaptic area is integrated across all collateral synapses of a single afferent. Functional surface area may reflect the amount of "release sites," for example, or the readily releasable store of neurotransmitter.

Presynaptic activity controls the dynamic aspect of Rule 3. Thus, the greater an afferent's average activity, the greater is its optimum amount of functional presynaptic surface area. For one afferent maintaining a constant, average level of activity, the total amount of functional surface area summed across all its synapses is limited to a single maximum value. If the afferent's activity increases, this value increases; if activity decreases, the value also decreases. Those afferents lacking their full complement of presynaptic territory are the ones most likely to participate in synaptogenesis.

Although afferents whose average activity has recently increased are obvious candidates for synaptogenesis, this need not be the case. Afferents with increased average activity may undergo sufficient proliferation of functional presynaptic surface area at existing synapses to maintain their optimum territory. Similarly, some afferents with an unchanged average level of activity may also participate in synaptogenesis (e.g., those afferents losing synaptic territory at other collateral synapses due to depression [excitatory rule 1b]).

In sum, excitatory rule 3 provides the basis for axonal growth regulated by excitatory rules 1a and 1b and by endogenous afferent activity. Excitatory rule 3 facilitates the formation of synaptic correlations, or associations, between afferents. However, afferents with many established synaptic correlations tend to not grow new synapses. Afferents of equivalent average activity with fewer or less potent synapses, on the other hand, do participate in axonal growth.

Further teleological motivation for this form of excitatory rule 3 arises from consideration of synaptogenesis without this rule. Without rule 3, presynaptic growth is random or based merely on spatial proximity between an afferent and a receptive postsynaptic cell. Nonspecific formulations of rule 3 might posit random growth by all afferents or the simplest form of trophic factor theory where the trophic factor induces afferent growth without regard to an afferent's activity or number of release sites.

A nonspecific rule 3 lacking activity-based specificity results in two unfavorable situations. First, synaptogenesis would not yield as much new information to correlate between afferents. Those afferents already innervating an inactive dendrite are not very useful, yet they have the most advantageous access, via random growth, to newly available postsynaptic sites. These same afferents would also receive the largest concentration of trophic factor. In neither case would synapse formation provide new correlations. Second, the redundant innervation resulting from random growth wastes free postsynaptic sites. Not only is it unlikely that the activity of these nearby afferents correlates with postsynaptic activity, but rule 1b does not remove this redundant innervation because insufficient postsynaptic activity exists to invoke the rule. A more useful afferent from which to obtain new information, and one that does not result in groups of identical clusters throughout the nervous system, is an afferent obeying rule 3.

Rule 2, in concert with rule 3, facilitates the formation of the maximum number of extant, but differing correlations, saving those unused (condition 1 of rule 2), confused (condition 2), and indecisive (condition 3) cells from a wasted existence. Rule 2 helps unused and indecisive neurons to form associations. Rule 3 provides the opportunity for afferents that are incompletely correlated relative to their activity levels to develop new correlations. Whether or not a postsynaptic structure, operating under the aforementioned conditions, can, by itself, stimulate synaptic proliferation via secretion of a trophic factor is important biologically, but not critical to the argument here. However, if trophic factors are secreted, an interactive decision process between pre- and postsynaptic structures seems advantageous for synapse formation.

Mathematical Embodiment of the Proposed Excitatory Rules

Excitatory Rules 1a and 1b: Hebb/anti-Hebb Rule.   For a particular moment of time,

$$\frac{dm_{ij}}{dt} = \epsilon \cdot f(y) \cdot (c_1 x_i - m_{ij})$$

where m_{ij} is the strength of the synapse formed by the ith afferent with the jth cell;

ϵ is a small number;

c_1 is a positive constant;

x_i is the firing frequency of the ith afferent; and

$f(y_j)$ is the net excitation of the postsynaptic structure.

The values of $f(y_j)$ are nonnegative (Levy & Steward, unpublished observations), increasing with increasing excitatory synaptic activation and decreasing with increasing inhibitory synaptic activation. Although the postsynaptic structure j is often spoken of as a cell, it is probably some portion of a cell (e.g., a dendritic segment). The linear assumption $f(y_j) = \Sigma m_{ij} x_i$ is often used and has simplicity in its favor. Of course, a binary function and more complicated continuous functions, such as those used by Cooper, Munro, and Scofield (chapter 9, this volume) are possible.

Changes in synaptic efficacy are related to the afferent firing frequency and synaptic strength. When $x_i > m_{ij}$, dm_{ij}/dt is positive, and the amount of potentiation increases in proportion to the amount of postsynaptic excitation $[f(\Sigma mx)]$. When the ith afferent fires at low frequency (i.e., when $x_i < m_{ij}$), the amount of depression at the synapse is also an increasing function of the amount of postsynaptic excitation $[f(\Sigma mx)]$.

Excitatory Rule 2: Postsynaptic Growth.   We propose two alternate forms of this rule. The first alternative is expressed in terms of the number of vacant postsynaptic sites; the more vacant sites a postsynaptic structure has, the more likely the postsynaptic structure will receive new innervation. This alternative could be equivalently formulated in terms of the amount of trophic factor secreted. Again, the idea is that the more trophic factor is secreted, the better the chances of the postsynaptic structure receiving new innervation. The first alternative takes the form of

$$\text{number of vacant sites on cell } j = \frac{c_2}{E[(y_j^P)] + c_3}$$

where c_2, c_3, and P are positive constants;

$E(\cdot)$ is an expected value; and

y_j is the net postsynaptic effect.

In the term y_j, active excitatory synapses are added linearly through their synaptic strengths while active inhibitory synapses are divisors scaled by frequency and synaptic strength. This formulation may be modified to accommodate subtractive inhibition.

Notice that in this equation, the number of vacant sites increases as postsynaptic activity decreases. In this scheme, the probability of new innervation increases in proportion to the number of vacant postsynaptic sites. As a convenience, excitatory rule 2 is expressed as a function of cell activity. Some smaller unit of integration (e.g., a dendritic segment) seems the more likely postsynaptic integrating unit.

The second alternative expression of excitatory rule 2 is formulated in terms of the total excitatory synaptic strength of the postsynaptic integrating unit. This equation is a dynamic formulation of von der Malsburg's (1973) suggestion that the sum of the synaptic strengths is a constant. This alternative form is

$$\sum_i m_{ij} = \frac{c_2}{E[(y_j^P)] + c_3}$$

All terms in this equation are as defined previously for excitatory rules 1 and 2. Note, however, that this alternative postsynaptic rule is summed over the ith afferents for one postsynaptic structure j.

Excitatory Rule 3: Axonal Growth.   There are two candidate forms of this excitatory rule. Both express a tendency for axonal growth with increased activity as tempered by the number (or amount) of extant synapses. The first alternative describes a boundary condition that constrains the system, whereas the second merely treats the system probabilistically. The boundary condition can be expressed as

$$\sum_j m_{ij} = c_4 E(x_i)$$

whereas the probabilistic expression is

$$\frac{c_4 E(x_i)}{\sum_j m_{ij}} = r_i$$

where c_4 is a positive constant;

$E(\cdot)$ is an expected value; and

i and j are as described previously.

In contrast to excitatory rule 2, which is summed over the ith afferents for one particular postsynaptic unit j, excitatory rule 3 is summed over the jth postsynaptic units for one particular afferent i.

The term r_i is a competitive factor for afferent i that expresses the relative probability of axonal growth. The larger the value of r, the better the particular afferent *i* will do in competition with homologous afferents for vacant postsynaptic sites.

Supporting Biological Data

Ample evidence (see Globus, 1975, for a general review) exists to support our basic premise that synaptic plasticity occurs in the mature nervous system, ranging from long-term potentiation within the hippocampal formation (Bliss & Lømo, 1973) to increases in cortical dendritic length and number following experience with an enriched environment (Juraska, Greenough, Elliott, Mack, & Berkowitz, 1980; Uylings, Kuypers, Diamond, & Veltman, 1978; Uylings, Kuypers, & Veltman, 1978) and perhaps with age in humans (Buell & Coleman, 1979, 1981).

Excitatory Rules 1a and 1b: Hebb/anti-Hebb Rule.   To explain learned perception, Hebb (1949) originally suggested that the synaptic efficacies of individual excitatory synapses might be adjusted as a function of the correlated activity between each synapse and the integrated activity of its target postsynaptic cell. Most critical to the performance of model neural systems and most critical for their correctness and relevance to brain function is the exact form of the Hebb rule. Our experimental work has concentrated on defining and demonstrating the elemental synaptic learning rule as it actually exists in the mammalian brain (see Levy, Chapter 1, this volume).

Synapses consistent with the Hebb/anti-Hebb rule have been characterized in the rat hippocampal formation (Levy & Steward, 1979) and proposed in kitten visual cortex (Rauschecker & Singer, 1979, 1981). A striking similarity exists between Rauschecker and Singer's explanation of the cellular mechanism subserving binocular competition and the associative potentiation/depression data of Levy and Steward (1979). In the entorhinal cortex–dentate gyrus system, convergent activity of the ipsilateral and crossed entorhinal inputs leads to enhanced synaptic efficacy in the dentate gyrus, whereas presynaptic inactivity during postsynaptic activity decreases synaptic efficacy (Levy & Steward, 1979). A change in ocular dominance in kitten visual cortex following monocular suture results from one input being inactive (sutured) while the other input is active (nonsutured) (Rauschecker & Singer, 1979, 1981). In other words, the competitive interaction between an afferent and its convergent, nearby neighbors depends on the form of the integrated postsynaptic excitation and is a function of the coactivity of each converging afferent. Two biological exemplars of the Hebb/anti-Hebb rule are thus well documented in the central nervous system.

Associative potentiation/depression receives substantial attention and some good experimental support in developing systems under rubrics such as competitive interactions, binocular competition, and selective stabilization (Changeux, chapter 5, this volume; Changeux & Danchin, 1976; Constantine-Paton & Law, 1978; Hebb, 1949; Law & Constantine-Paton, 1980, 1981; LeVay, Wiesel, & Hubel, 1980; Pittman & Oppenheim, 1979; Sargent & Dennis, 1981).

We have been purposely vague about the nature of the postsynaptic element involved in the synaptic learning rule. The postsynaptic unit could be localized regions of dendritic excitation or postsynaptic cell firing. Unambiguous definition of the form of $f(y)$ is difficult, especially as the postsynaptic event permitting potentiation/depression may be localized to particular dendritic zones (Levy & Steward, in preparation). Therefore, the efferent activity of the postsynaptic cell does not necessarily reflect the relevant variable for plasticity. During conditioning stimulation, for example, localized forms of inhibition might inhibit postsynaptic cell firing but would be substantially irrelevant to the primary regions of synaptic activation.

Excitatory Rule 2: Postsynaptic Growth.   Excitatory rule 2 permits new synapses to grow only when the activity of the postsynaptic integrating unit is low. On the other hand, when postsynaptic activity is high, the number of vacant synaptic sites is practically zero, and little postsynaptic growth occurs. Whether or not trophic factors are released by the postsynaptic cell is not critical to this theory. However, increased release of trophic factors with inactivity is consistent with the overall concept of excitatory rule 2.

Even though the intuitive perspectives of Ariens Kappers (1921) and Hebb (1949) yield the notion that postsynaptic activity is a stimulus for the formation of new synapses, inactivity is a more useful trigger for synaptic proliferation. Inactivity as the stimulus ensures maximum utilization of all cells while avoiding the formation of cells that are active in the extreme. This perspective does not, however, eliminate the importance of postsynaptic activity. As soon as innervation occurs, the competitive synaptic principles of associative potentiation/depression, in part ruled by some form of postsynaptic excitation, assume control of synapse survival.

Although counterintuitive from Hebb's (1949) viewpoint, data from peripheral synapses support the notion of a dynamic constant. At the neuromuscular junction, denervation-induced supersensitivity has been known for years. Preeminent is the work of Lømo and colleagues (Lømo, 1980, Lømo & Slater, 1978) who demonstrated experimentally that additional and new innervation of adult muscle depends on and requires postsynaptic inactivity. Junctional inactivity leads to a surface membrane receptive to new innervation (Fex, Sonesson, Thesleff, & Zelena, 1966; Lømo & Rosenthal, 1972; Miledi, 1963). Moreover, successful hyperinnervation of the rat soleus muscle depends on muscle inactivity (Jansen, Lømo, Nicolaysen, & Westgaard, 1973).

In nervous tissue, an experiment by Wolff, Joo, Dames, and Feher (1979) provides the strongest evidence for the inverse relationship between receptivity for new innervation and postsynaptic activity. Treating the adult superior cervical ganglion with an inhibitory neurotransmitter, γ-aminobutyric acid (GABA), leads to the appearance of postsynaptic junctional densities at extrasynaptic dendritic loci, as well as increased extrasynaptic surface of the ganglion cells. Because GABA application to the superior cervical ganglion suppresses presynaptic action potentials, GABA (though probably not usually present) inhibits dendritic activity of the ganglion cells. The formation of extrasynaptic postsynaptic densities supports the notion that inactive dendrites are receptive to new innervation.

The work of Wolff et al. (1979) suggests a mechanism that might be operative in the dentate gyrus. Namely, large amounts of GABA-mediated inhibition may yield postsynaptic cells receptive to new innervation.

The second alternative form of excitatory rule 2, that the total excitatory strength of the postsynaptic integrating unit is a constant, has an experimental prediction about synaptic shedding not explicit in the rule's first form. It may seem that excitatory rule 1b can account for the shedding of synapses. Actually, this rule only predicts that a synapse asymptotically approaches the value of zero without ever reaching zero as long as the afferent making the synaptic contact maintains a minimum noise level of activity. In the second formulation of excitatory rule 2, the competitive idea of excitatory rule 1b is extended to its ultimate manifestation.

Data supporting the second form of excitatory rule 2 comes from a study of associative potentiation/depression in the dentate gyrus (Desmond & Levy, 1983, Levy & Desmond, in preparation). Following conditioning stimulation of the entorhinal afferents to the dentate gyrus, synaptic density increases not within the region of the dentate molecular layer receiving the greatest synaptic excitation, but within the regions bordering the zone of maximal synaptic activation. This localized increase in synaptic density is interpreted as synaptic proliferation triggered by postsynaptic inactivity surrounding a central band of excitation. Given the well-known distribution of GABAergic synapses in the dentate molecular layer (Nadler, White, Vaca, & Cotman, 1977; Palacios, Wamsley, & Kuhar, 1981; Ribak, Vaughn, & Saito, 1978), disynaptic inhibition may result from entorhinal activation such that outside the central lamina of active synapses, there is net inhibition. These dendritic regions consistently receiving net inhibition prepare sites for synaptic attachment at which "prototype" synapses are induced.

Excitatory Rule 3: Axonal Growth.   The activity dependence of excitatory rule 3 stands in distinct contrast to excitatory rule 2. Although both rules exert control over new synapse formation, they govern opposite sides of the synapse and do so in quite opposite ways. That is, their dynamic dependencies are reversed, with axonal growth of an input becoming more energetic as that afferent's average activity increases. In contrast, postsynaptic targets, according to excitatory rule 2, become more receptive to new innervation as their activity decreases.

The evidence that axons can find new synaptic connections is quite abundant for the mature nervous system. When one input to a structure is lesioned, a second input normally innervating that structure extends its axons to occupy dendrites previously contacted by the lesioned axons. This sprouting phenomenon has been demonstrated in a variety of CNS regions, including spinal cord (Bernstein & Bernstein, 1967, 1969), red nucleus (Tsukahara, 1978), septum (Raisman, 1969), and hippocampus (Cotman & Nadler, 1978). Results of complex environment experiments (Greenough, 1976) also support the contention that axons extend to form novel synaptic contacts.

Bernstein and Bernstein (1967) are among the first to suggest that the amount or number of synapses an axon possesses limits its tendency to grow and develop further synapses. Experiments in the peripheral and central nervous systems support this idea, suggesting that an afferent can only maintain a limited number of synapses (however, cf. Jansen et al., 1973). In the Bixby and Van Essen (1979) study of peripheral nervous system, transplanting a nerve to a normally innervated skeletal muscle results in the proliferation of new synapses and the loss of old synapses. In later developmental stages of the central visual system, lesions that remove one target tissue of an afferent result in the proliferation of that same afferent in other regions (Schneider, 1973). These studies show that limits are placed on the extent of an afferent field. Whether or not this value is dynamically regulated is an experimental question. If afferents are generally near their maximum allowable size, then synaptic proliferation experiments require dynamic regulation, e.g., studies producing synaptogenesis with electrical stimulation (Rutledge, 1978; Levy & Desmond, in preparation).

The influence of the activity level of these axons remains unexplored. Excitatory rule 3 posits that highly active axons may search for novel synaptic connections or become particularly sensitive to trophic factors released by target neurons. A study using electrical stimulation to increase presynaptic activity and thereby improve reinnervation of a lesioned structure would provide good experimental support for excitatory rule 3. However, care would be required to ensure that postsynaptic activity is not altered when performing the study so that the results can be interpreted strictly relative to this rule.

Certainly, however, rules 2 and 3 are very specific in their predictions for regrowth in the mature sprouting system where sprouting is often incomplete. These rules suggest that a greater amount of synaptogenesis can be obtained with concurrent pharmacological inhibition of the target cells and stimulation of the sprouting axons.

The great similarity between the rules presented here and the rules postulated to account for neural development is not likely to be by chance. For instance, axonal extension and dendritic shedding are issues in developmental neurobiology (see, e.g., the selective stabilization hypothesis of Changeux &

Danchin, 1976, the dynamic equilibrium hypothesis of Young, 1951, and Vaughn & Sims', 1978 study of synapse development).

The fact that these rules are not limited to any particular stage of an animal's life is intentional. The well-known differences in synaptic plasticity with age need not be attributed to aging of the enzymatic machinery or cellular DNA. Rather, the reduced plasticity of older animals may simply reflect the fact that the overall environment is highly regular and that most cells and synapses are near their prescribed equilibrium values.

INHIBITORY SYNAPSES

This section on inhibitory synapses is necessarily brief because, compared with excitatory synapses, there are little data from which to conceptualize the modification rules for inhibitory synapses. This is not to say that inhibitory synapses lack plasticity with time and/or use. Not only does intuition argue that Nature would not waste 15% of the cerebral cortical synapses, but experiments certainly exist showing inhibitory synaptic plasticity. The problem with these experiments is that it is unclear just what the correlated and noncorrelated activity of the pre- and postsynaptic cells are. Experiments demonstrating inhibitory modifications include Rutledge (1978), Liebowitz, Pedley, and Cutler (1978), McNamara, Peper, & Patrone (1980), Nadler (1981), and Valdes, Dasheiff, Birmingham, Crutcher, & McNamara (1982). These studies involve very gross manipulations such as lesions or daily electrical stimulations with unknown, diffuse, and complex responses of the inhibitory cells. These inhibitory neurons are presumably interneurons and therefore are not monosynaptically activated by the conditioning stimulations.

The Postulated Rules

Because we cannot rely on physiology to direct us as we did for the excitatory synaptic modification rules, there is only intuition as a guide. In this case intuition is shaped by two elements: (1) the framework already provided by the rules for excitatory synaptic modification; and (2) our attempts (Levy, in preparation) to construct neural models that perform realistically within various aspects of the classical conditioning paradigm as well as models that give responses based on conditional probabilities.

For these two modeling problems, the noncorrelation of input active–output silent must be encoded. Excitatory rule 1b encodes the other noncorrelation event (i.e., input silent–output active [*vide supra*]). Although Cooper et al. (1979) prefer to incorporate the input active–output inactive noncorrelation in their model at excitatory synapses, our solution is to encode this required noncorrelation at inhibitory synapses.

The inhibitory rules that follow refer to the conditions leading to synaptic alterations for inhibitory synapses:

1a. Presynaptic activity paired with postsynaptic inactivity leads to potentiation at the active inhibitory synapse.

1b. Postsynaptic activity should be required for a loss of strength of the inhibitory synapse. Three forms of this rule have been found satisfactory: (1) postsynaptic activity without presynaptic inactivity; (2) postsynaptic activity with presynaptic activity; and (3) both (1) and (2).

2. Postsynaptic activity increases the receptivity of the postsynaptic cell for new inhibitory innervation.

3. The limits of presynaptic growth increase with increasing presynaptic activity and decrease with decreasing presynaptic activity.

Mathematical Embodiment of the Proposed Inhibitory Rules

Inhibitory Rules 1a and 1b. Depending on the anatomical inter-relationships assumed and the system performance desired, one of the following three alternative forms of inhibitory rule 1 are suitable for constructing systems that produce conditional probabilities, conditional odds, and likelihood ratios. The respective equations, for a particular moment of time, are:

$$\frac{dl_{ij}}{dt} = \epsilon_2 \cdot (c_5 x_i - y_j l_{ij}) ,$$

$$\frac{dl_{ij}}{dt} = \epsilon_2 c_6 x_i - \epsilon_2 y_j (c_5 x_i + l_{ij}) ,$$

and

$$\frac{dl_{ij}}{dt} = \epsilon_2 y_j (E(x_i) - x_i - c_5 l_{ij})$$

where l_{ij} is the strength of the inhibitory synapse formed by the *ith* afferent with the *jth* cell;

ϵ_2 is a small number;

c_5 and c_6 are positive constants;

x_i is the firing frequency of the *ith* afferent;

y_j is the net excitation of the postsynaptic unit; and

$E(x_i)$ is the expected value of x_i.

We have assumed a linear relationship between y_j and $\sum_i l_{ij} x_i$; however, this need not be the case.

A third equation is suitable for combination with excitatory rule 1 to build a system that mimics the classical conditioning paradigm, including extinction and blocking:

$$\frac{dl_{ij}}{dt} = \epsilon_2 c_5 x_i (l - c_6 y_j)$$

Inhibitory Rules 2 and 3. Two alternative forms of each of these inhibitory rules exist. In the interest of brevity, each rule is presented in only one form. However, the alternative forms that parallel the alternatives of excitatory rules 2 and 3 should be given equal consideration.

For inhibitory rule 2,

$$\frac{\text{number of vacant inhibitory}}{\text{postsynaptic sites on cell } j} = \frac{c_7 E(y_j^p)}{\sum_i l_{ij} + c_8}$$

whereas inhibitory rule 3 is summed over the *jth* postsynaptic units for one particular afferent *i*.

Teleology

Inhibitory Rules 1a and 1b. The importance of inhibitory rules 1a and 1b has already been indicated for learning responses based on conditional probabilities and for the extinction portion of the classical conditioning paradigm. In addition, encoding this form of noncorrelation (input active–output silent) is required to explain those aspects of visual development modeled by Cooper et al. (this volume).

Inhibitory Rules 2 and 3. Inhibitory rules 2 and 3 provide for the formation of new inhibitory synapses and are formulated in the same vein as excitatory rules 2 and 3. However, in contrast to excitatory rule 2, highly active cells are more likely to receive new inhibitory information than are less active cells. Just like excitatory rule 3, the more active inhibitory presynaptic afferents are those with the most available information and are more likely to establish new synapses.

Finally, we should point out an essential difference between some excitatory and inhibitory connections. The existence of multiple synaptic contacts on one cell seems rare for many types of excitatory afferents, but often seems the rule for inhibitory afferents. In addition, in many systems inhibitory neurons are greatly outnumbered by excitatory cells and the number of excitatory afferents. It may be that inhibitory systems are much more coarsely modulated than are excitatory systems. Thus, rather than three separate inhibitory modification rules, there might be only one rule that has the same net effect as the three rules, but merely modulates synapse number rather than the strength of individual inhibitory synapses. The properties of this one inhibitory rule should, however, resemble the properties of the three individual rules proposed here.

ACKNOWLEDGMENT

The work described in this chapter was supported in part by NIH grant NS15488 to William B. Levy.

REFERENCES

Amari, S. I. Neural theory of association and concept-formation. *Biol. Cybernetics*, 1977, *26*, 175–185.

Anderson, J. A. A memory storage model utilizing spatial correlation functions. *Kybernetik*, 1968, *5*, 113–119.

Anderson, J. A. Parallel computation with simple neural networks. *Cognition & Brain Theory*, 1979, *3*, 45–53.

Ariens Kappers, C. U. On the structural laws in the nervous system: The principles of neurobiotaxis. *Brain*, 1921, *44*, 125–149.

Bernstein, J. J., & Bernstein, M. E. Effect of glial-ependymal scar and teflon arrest on the regenerative capacity in goldfish spinal cord. *Exp. Neurol.*, 1967, *19*, 25–32.

Bernstein, J. J., & Bernstein, M. E. Ultrastructure of normal regeneration and loss of regenerative capacity following teflon blockage in goldfish spinal cord. *Exp. Neurol.*, 1969, *24*, 538–557.

Bixby, J. L., & Van Essen, D. C. Competition between foreign and original nerves in adult mammalian skeletal muscle. *Nature*, 1979, *282*, 726–728.

Bliss, T. V. P., & Lømo, T. Long-lasting potentiation of synaptic transmission in the dentate area of the anaesthetized rabbit following stimulation of the perforant path. *J. Physiol.*, 1973, *232*, 331–356.

Buell, S. J., & Coleman, P. D. Dendritic growth in the aged human brain and failure of growth in senile dementia. *Science*, 1979, *206*, 854–856.

Buell, S. J., & Coleman, P. D. Quantitative evidence for selective dendritic growth in normal human aging but not in senile dementia. *Brain Res.*, 1981, *214*, 23–41.

Changeux, J.-P., & Danchin, A. Selective stabilisation of developing synapses as a mechanism for the specification of neuronal networks. *Nature*, 1976, *264*, 705–712.

Constantine-Paton, M., & Law, M. Eye-specific termination bands in the tecta of three-eyed frogs. *Science*, 1978, *202*, 639–641.

Cooper, L. N., Liberman, F., & Oja, E. A theory for the acquisition and loss of neuron specificity in visual cortex. *Biol. Cybernetics*, 1979, *33*, 9–28.

Cotman, C. W., & Nadler, J. V. Reactive synaptogenesis in the hippocampus. In C. W. Cotman (Ed.), *Neuronal plasticity*. New York: Raven Press, 1978.

Desmond, N. L., & Levy, W. B. Synaptic correlates of associative potentiation/depression: An ultrastructural study in the hippocampus. *Brain Res.*, 1983, *265*, 21–30.

Fex, S., Sonesson, B., Thesleff, S., & Zelena, J. Nerve implants in botulinum poisoned mammalian muscle. *J. Physiol.*, 1966, *184*, 872–882.

Globus, A. Brain morphology as a function of presynaptic morphology and activity. In A. H. Riesen (Ed.), *The developmental neuropsychology of sensory deprivation*. New York: Academic Press, 1975.

Greenough, W. T. Enduring brain effects of differential experience and training. In M. R. Rosenzweig & E. L. Bennett (Eds.), *Neural mechanisms of learning and memory*. Cambridge, Mass.: MIT Press, 1976.

Hebb, D. O. *The organization of behavior*. New York: Wiley, 1949.

Jansen, J. K. S., Lømo, T., Nicolaysen, K., & Westgaard, R. H. Hyperinnervation of skeletal muscle fibers: Dependence on muscle activity. *Science*, 1973, *181*, 559–561.

Juraska, J. M., Greenough, W. T., Elliott, C., Mack, K. J., & Berkowitz, R. Plasticity in adult rat visual cortex: An examination of several cell populations after differential rearing. *Behav. Neural. Biol.*, 1980, *29*, 157–167.

Kohonen, T. *Correlation matrix memories*. Report TKK–F–A130. Espoo, Finland: Helsinki University of Technology, 1970.

Kohonen, T. *Associative memory. A system–theoretical approach*. New York: Springer Verlag, 1977.

Kohonen, T., Lehtio, P., & Rovano, J. Modelling of neural associative memory. *Ann. Acad. Scient. Fenn. A. V. Med.*, 1974, *167*, 1–18.

Law, M., & Constantine-Paton, M. Right and left eye bands in frogs with unilateral tectal ablations. *Proc. Natl. Acad. Sci. USA*, 1980, *77*, 2314–2318.

Law, M. I., & Constantine-Paton, M. Anatomy and physiology of experimentally produced striped tecta. *J. Neurosci.*, 1981, *1*, 741–759.

LeVay, S., Wiesel, T. N., & Hubel, D. H. The development of ocular dominance columns in normal and visually deprived monkeys. *J. Comp. Neurol.*, 1980, *191*, 1–51.

Levy, W. B., & Steward, O. Synapses as associative memory elements in the hippocampal formation. *Brain Res.*, 1979, *175*, 233–245.

Liebowitz, N. R., Pedley, T. A., & Cutler, R. W. P. Release of γ-aminobutyric acid from hippocampal slices of the rat following generalized seizures induced by daily electrical stimulation of entorhinal cortex. *Brain Res.*, 1978, *138*, 369–373.

Lømo, T. The role of impulse activity in the formation of neuromuscular junctions. In J. Taxi (Ed.), *Ontogenesis and functional mechanisms of peripheral synapses*. Amsterdam: Elsevier, 1980.

Lømo, T., & Rosenthal, J. Control of ACh sensitivity by muscle activity in the rat. *J. Physiol.*, 1972, *221*, 493–513.

Lømo, T., & Slater, C. R. Control of acetylcholine sensitivity and synapse formation by muscle activity. *J. Physiol.*, 1978, *275*, 391–402.

Marr, D. Simple memory: A theory for archicortex. *Phil. Trans. Roy. Soc. Lond. B*, 1971, *262*, 23–81.

McNamara, J. O., Peper, A. M., & Patrone, V. Repeated seizures induce long-term increase in hippocampal benzodiazepine receptors. *Proc. Natl. Acad. Sci. USA*, 1980, *77*, 3029–3032.

Miledi, R. Formation of extra nerve-muscle junctions in innervated muscle. *Nature*, 1963, *199*, 1191–1192.

Nadler, J. V. Desensitization-like changes in GABA receptor binding of rat fascia dentata after entorhinal lesion. *Neurosci. Lett.*, 1981, *26*, 275–281.

Nadler, J. V., White, W. F., Vaca, K. W., & Cotman, C. W. Calcium-dependent γ-aminobutyrate release by interneurons of rat hippocampal regions: Lesion-induced plasticity. *Brain Res.*, 1977, *131*, 241–258.

Palacios, J. M., Wamsley, J. K., & Kuhar, M. J. High affinity GABA receptors — autoradiographic localization. *Brain Res.*, 1981, *222*, 285–307.

Pittman, R., & Oppenheim, R. W. Cell death of motoneurons in the chick embryo spinal cord. IV. Evidence that a functional neuromuscular interaction is involved in the regulation of naturally occurring cell death and the stabilization of synapses. *J. Comp. Neurol.*, 1979, *187*, 425–446.

Raisman, G. Neuronal plasticity in the septal nuclei of the adult rat. *Brain Res.*, 1969, *14*, 25–48.

Ramon y Cajal, S. *Histologie du système nerveux de l'homme et des vertébrés*. Paris: A. Maloine, 1911.

Ranck, J. B., Jr. Synaptic "learning" due to electroosmosis: A theory. *Science*, 1964, *144*, 187–189.

Rauschecker, J. P., & Singer, W. Changes in the circuitry of the kitten visual cortex are gated by postsynaptic activity. *Nature*, 1979, *280*, 58–60.

Rauschecker, J. P., & Singer, W. The effects of early visual experience on the cat's visual cortex and their possible explanation by Hebb synapses. *J. Physiol.*, 1981, *310*, 215-239.

Ribak, C. E., Vaughn, J. E., & Saito, K. Immunocytochemical localization of glutamic acid decarboxylase in neuronal somata following colchicine inhibition of axonal transport. *Brain Res.*, 1978, *140*, 315-332.

Rosenblatt, F. Recent work on theoretical models of biological memory. In J. T. Tou (Ed.), *Computer and information sciences-II.* New York: Academic Press, 1967.

Rutledge, L. T. The effects of denervation and stimulation upon synaptic ultrastructure. *J. Comp. Neurol.*, 1978, *178*, 117-128.

Sargent, P. B., & Dennis, M. J. The influence of normal innervation upon abnormal synaptic connections between frog parasympathetic neurons. *Develop. Biol.*, 1981, *81*, 65-73.

Schneider, G. E. Early lesions of superior colliculus: Factors affecting the formation of abnormal retinal projections. *Brain, Behav. Evol.*, 1973, *8*, 73-109.

Stent, G. S. A physiological mechanism for Hebb's postulate of learning. *Proc. Natl. Acad. Sci. USA*, 1973, *70*, 997-1001.

Tsukahara, N. Synaptic plasticity in the red nucleus. In C. W. Cotman (Ed.), *Neuronal plasticity*. New York: Raven Press, 1978.

Uttley, A. M. Neurophysiological predictions of a two-pathway informon theory of neural conditioning. *Brain Res.*, 1976, *102*, 55-70. (a)

Uttley, A. M. Simulation studies of learning in an informon network. *Brain Res.*, 1976, *102*, 37-53. (b)

Uttley, A. M. A two-pathway informon theory of conditioning and adaptive pattern recognition. *Brain Res.*, 1976, *102*, 23-35. (c)

Uylings, H. B. M., Kuypers, K., Diamond, M. C., & Veltman, W. A. M. Effects of differential environments on plasticity of dendrites of cortical pyramidal neurons in adult rats. *Exp. Neurol.*, 1978, *62*, 658-677.

Uylings H. B. M., Kuypers, K., & Veltman, W. A. M. Environmental influences in the neocortex in later life. *Prog. Brain Res.*, 1978, *48*, 261-274.

Valdes, F., Dasheiff, R. M., Birmingham, F., Crutcher, K. A., & McNamara, J. O. Benzodiazepine receptor increases after repeated seizures: Evidence for localization to dentate granule cells. *Proc. Natl. Acad. Sci. USA*, 1982, *79*, 193-197.

Vaughn, J. E., & Sims, T. J. Axonal growth cones and developing axonal collaterals form synaptic junctions in embryonic mouse spinal cord. *J. Neurocytol.*, 1978, *7*, 337-363.

von der Malsburg, C. Self-organization of orientation sensitive cells in the striate cortex. *Kybernetik*, 1973, *14*, 85-100.

Wolff, J. R., Joo, F., Dames, W., & Feher, O. Induction and maintenance of free postsynaptic membrane thickenings in the adult superior cervical ganglion. *J. Neurocytol.*, 1979, *8*, 549-563.

Young, J. Z. Growth and plasticity in the nervous system. *Proc. Roy. Soc. Lond. B*, 1951, *139*, 18-37.

7 Neural Problem Solving

Andrew G. Barto
Richard S. Sutton
Department of Computer and Information Science
University of Massachusetts

Neural models, and indeed models in any domain, can differ widely in terms of the intentions with which they are constructed and the levels of empirical support on which they depend. A neural model might be based on detailed observations of a particular experimental preparation, or it may be less directly related to anatomical and physiological data, relying instead on behavioral parallels. As neural models become farther removed from anatomy and physiology and closer to "adaptive networks" or "self-organizing systems" of quasi-neural elements, they become less interesting to the neuroscientist, and the term "neural model" becomes more misleading. With this decreasing relevance to neuroscience, however, one might hope for increasing relevance to psychology and perhaps to artificial intelligence. Yet many such models have not been influential among psychologists despite the rich history in psychology of purely descriptive behavioral models, and they have not been influential among artificial intelligence researchers despite the fact that these researchers have explicitly excluded concern with neural mechanisms. One reason for this may be the fact that many abstract neural models neither make significant contact with behavioral data nor suggest algorithms that would be useful to the artificial intelligence researcher for solving nontrivial problems.

In this article, we present an overview of a research program that is intended explicitly to be a study of "adaptive networks" of quasi-neural elements. However, we have tried to maintain careful and significant contact with behavioral data from animal learning studies, with descriptive behavioral models in that field, and with problem-solving methods of artificial intelligence. Although the mechanisms we discuss can be given neural interpretations, we feel that it is premature to propose an extensive and detailed neural model to bridge the gap between anatomical and physiological data and the behavioral level in which we are interested. We have instead concentrated on behavioral models that exhibit aspects of animal behavior that we consider to be adaptively significant, and on the relationship between these aspects of behavior and the computational requirements for solving nontrivial problems. We are considering problems that animals are capable of solving routinely, whose solutions provide obvious adaptive advantages, and that are genuinely difficult to solve irrespective of the methods used.

Our approach is to consider the general problem of *control*. Arbib (1972) emphasizes that: "the animal perceives its environment to the extent that it is *prepared* to *interact* with that environment in some reasonably structured fashion." This stress on what Arbib calls "action oriented perception" implies that modeling approaches are misleading insofar as they consider just sensory processing (e.g., pattern recognition), while neglecting highly structured action generation processes and the closed-loop interaction, mediated by the organism's environment, between action and sensory patterns. From an engineering point of view, we can say that animals are engaged in the problem of controlling their environments in a closed-loop fashion to achieve certain goals. Consequently, our strategy has been to consider entire control systems facing control problems posed by environmental interaction, and we have paid as much attention to the environments and the resulting control problems as we have to the controlling mechanisms themselves.

In addition to our emphasis on complete control problems, we have found it useful to endow each network component with relatively sophisticated computational power. Each primitive component of a network in our approach is best characterized as a complete, although simple, "reinforcement learning control system" (Mendel & McLaren, 1970) that acquires knowledge about feedback pathways in which it is embedded and uses this knowledge to seek preferred inputs. In providing each component with such capabilities, we have been guided by the proposal of A. H. Klopf (1972, 1979, 1982) that progress in understanding natural intelligence, and progress in artificial intelligence, might be furthered by a study of goal-seeking systems composed of goal-seeking components. Instead of viewing any form of goal-seeking behavior as an emergent property of a system consisting of non–goal-seeking components, Klopf suggests that sophisticated goal-directed behavior arises from interacting components that are self-interested, and exercise strategies for furthering these self-interests. Goal-directed behavior is pushed down the structural hierarchy to basic levels, and higher forms of goal-directed behavior are seen as resulting from the competitive and cooperative interaction of self-interested components. The neural interpretation of this hypothesis is that neurons are similarly sophisticated goal-seeking control systems. In the course of our discussion, we point out similarities between our adaptive elements and goal-seeking strategies known to exist in single-celled organisms such as bacteria. We think that the continued study of the numerous commonalities between bacterial chemotaxis and other simple forms of adaptive behavior in single cells, and the signaling systems of neurons (Koshland, 1979) is a most promising avenue for assessing the hypothesis that neurons are goal-seeking control systems. However, although we present our learning algorithms in terms of neuronlike elements, we are not prepared to argue that all the capabilities of these elements need necessarily reside at the level of single cells.

This article is divided into three major parts. In the first part, we discuss a neuronlike adaptive element that is capable of reproducing some of the details of animal behavior in classical conditioning experiments. We emphasize aspects of classical conditioning that are difficult to achieve by neural models proposed in the past and that seem to have obvious adaptive significance; in particular, we emphasize temporal phenomena involving prediction and expectation. This adaptive element resulted from our attempts to incorporate the sensitivity to temporal succession that seems necessary for goal-seeking control: If actions are to be selected according to their consequences, then temporal factors are important because an action's consequences unfold over time. This adaptive element is not, however, capable of closed-loop control and is not a goal-seeking system in the appropriate sense. In the second part of this article, another type of adaptive element is discussed that is a goal-seeking learning control system closely related to instrumental, rather than to classical, conditioning. We discuss associative networks composed of these elements, how their capabilities differ from associative memories studied in the past, and why these differences are important from a problem-solving perspective. We illustrate the learning capabilities of these networks in several spatial learning tasks. Finally, in the third section, we discuss how the open-loop classical conditioning element and the closed-loop goal-seeking element can interact to provide an approach to a fundamental problem of adaptive system theory known as the "assignment of credit problem": If reward is achieved after a complex series of actions, to which component actions should the credit be assigned (or the blame in the case of penalty)?

ANALOGS OF CLASSICAL CONDITIONING

Many adaptive network theories are based on neuronlike adaptive elements that can behave as single unit analogs of animal classical conditioning (e.g., elements incorporating Hebb's, 1949, postulate). However, there are many features of animal behavior in classical conditioning experiments that are generally not preserved by adaptive element analogs. Although one may validly question the rationale for investigating networks of elements that are *ex-*

act analogs of overt animal associative learning behavior (as surely some properties of this behavior must be due to the effects of higher levels of organization), it seems reasonable to include those characteristics that are most salient in terms of adaptive significance, that are problematic to achieve as emergent properties of organizations of simpler components, and that offer advantages from a problem-solving point of view. Here we describe an adaptive element analog of classical conditioning that preserves features of the anticipatory nature of classical conditioning and is in agreement with data regarding the effects of stimulus context in classical conditioning. We show that these stimulus context effects can be interpreted as the capability to "orthogonalize" input vectors. The element is a temporally refined extension of the Rescorla–Wagner model of classical conditioning (Rescorla & Wagner, 1972) and was presented by Sutton and Barto (1981b) and further discussed by Barto and Sutton (1982).

In a simple classical conditioning experiment, the subject is repeatedly presented with a neutral conditioned stimulus (CS), that is, a stimulus that does not cause responses other than orienting responses, followed after an interval of time (the interstimulus interval, or ISI) by an unconditioned stimulus (UCS), which reflexively causes an unconditioned response (UCR). After a number of such pairings of the CS and the UCS–UCR, the CS comes to elicit a response of its own, the conditioned response (CR), which closely resembles the UCR or some part of it. For example, a dog is repeatedly presented with first the sound of a bell (the CS) and then food (the UCS), which causes the dog to salivate (the UCR). Eventually, just the sound of the bell causes salivation (the CR). This description leaves much unsaid, as we see later, but will suffice as we describe an adaptive element analog.

Fig. 7.1 shows an adaptive element with an input pathway for the UCS and one for each stimulus capable of being associated with the UCS. These latter stimuli are (potential) conditioned stimuli, and we denote them by CS_i, $1 \leq i \leq n$. Let $x_0(t)$ denote the activity of the UCS pathway at time t, and let $x_i(t)$ denote the activity of pathway CS_i, $1 \leq i \leq n$, at time t. The element's output is assumed to contribute to both the UCR and the CR. For our present purposes, we assume that these activity levels at any time are positive real numbers. The associative strength of each CS at time t with respect to the UCS is denoted by $V_{CS_i}(t)$, $1 \leq i \leq n$, and represents the efficacy, or weight, of the corresponding input pathway. The weight of the UCS pathway is fixed at some constant value that we denote by λ. Let $s(t)$ denote the weighted sum of all the inputs at time t, that is,

$$s(t) = \lambda x_0(t) + \sum_{i=1}^{n} V_{CS_i}(t)x_i(t). \tag{1}$$

For our present purposes, it does not matter exactly how the element output is computed, and for simplicity, we assume that at time t it is just $s(t)$.

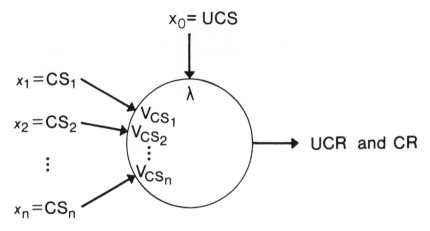

FIG. 7.1   An adaptive element analog of classical conditioning. (Reprinted from Barto & Sutton, 1982).

Several other variables are required in order to define the adaptive element. For each stimulus signal x_i, $1 \leq i \leq n$, we require a separate stimulus trace that we denote by $\bar{x}_i$. By this we mean that activity of variable x_i is reflected in later activity of variable $\bar{x}_i$. This is accomplished by letting $\bar{x}_i(t)$ be a weighted average of the values of x_i for some period of time preceding t. Similarly, we require a trace of the sum s. Let $\bar{s}(t)$ denote a weighted average of the values of s over some interval preceding t. In the computer simulations described as follows, we generated these traces using the first-order linear difference equations

$$\bar{x}_i(t + 1) = \alpha \bar{x}_i(t) + (1 - \alpha)x_i(t)$$
$$\bar{s}(t + 1) = \beta \bar{s}(t) + (1 - \beta)s(t)$$

where α and β are constants such that $0 \leq \alpha$, $\beta < 1$. This process produces exponentially decaying traces with time constants depending on the parameters α and β (Fig. 7.2).

In terms of the two variables s and $\bar{s}$, and the variables x_i, $\bar{x}_i$, and V_{CS_i} for each pathway $1 \leq i \leq n$, the adaptive element successively generates values of the associative strengths, or weights, as follows: for each i, $1 \leq i \leq n$,

$$V_{CS_i}(t + 1) = V_{CS_i}(t) + c[s(t) - \bar{s}(t)]\bar{x}_i(t) \tag{2}$$

where c is a positive constant determining the rate of learning.

The process specified by Equations 1 and 2 can be described as follows: Activity on any input pathway i possibly causes an immediate change in the element output s (we have assumed, again for simplicity, that there is no delay through the element) and also causes that pathway to be "tagged" by the

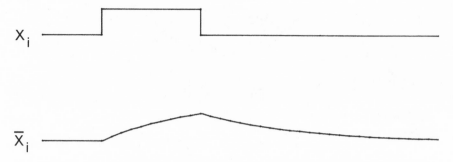

FIG. 7.2   An exponentially decaying stimulus trace. Activity of variable x_i causes a prolonged trace $\bar{x}_i$.

stimulus trace $\bar{x}_i$ as being "eligible" for modification for a certain period of time (the duration of the trace) after the activity on pathway i ceases. A weight is modified only if it is eligible and the current value of s differs from the value of the trace $\bar{s}$ of s. The simplest case, and the one used in our simulations, results from letting $\bar{s}(t) = s(t - 1)$ so that $s(t) - \bar{s}(t) = s(t) - s(t - 1)$, which is a discrete form of the rate of change of s.

The notion that one set of conditions makes pathway efficacies "eligible" for modification, but that actual modifications occur due to other conditions during periods of eligibility, is a major feature of Klopf's (1972, 1982) theory of neural adaptation. This notion itself is not uncommon among theorists, but the idea of two separate variables, one for signaling the occurrence of events and another for retaining knowledge of these occurrences so that events can be associated with later events, has not been deeply explored. In many neural theories, for example, neural discharges signal the occurrence of stimulus events and also bridge the temporal gap required for conditioning by "reverberating" in some manner. Because it seems advantageous for an organism to be able to perceive events as occurring as closely as possible to their actual times of occurrence, and particularly as early as possible, additional mechanisms must be postulated to distinguish neural activity that is signaling the occurrence of an event from reverberatory neural activity that is storing reflections of past events. In a two-variable system (e.g., x_i and $\bar{x}_i$) these two functions are cleanly separated. Although reverberatory activity is probably important at many levels in the central nervous system, one need not assume that reverberation is the primary mechanism at all levels for spanning the time between the sequential events on which learning depends. We now examine several aspects of our adaptive element's behavior with respect to classical conditioning data and suggest how these aspects of behavior are important from the perspective of problem solving.

Anticipatory Nature of Classical Conditioning

The interval between CS onset and CR onset is called the *CR latency*. For a particular response there is a positive minimum CR latency due to various types of intrinsic delays (e.g., 70–80 msec for rabbit nictitating-membrane response). If the ISI in a conditioning experiment is shorter than the minimum CR latency, then the CR necessarily begins after UCS onset. More usually, however, the ISI is longer than the minimum CR latency, and the CR begins before the UCS onset (although the CR latency tends to change during conditioning procedures [see, for example, Kimmell, 1965]). Being a response to the predictive CS, the CR *anticipates* the UCS and the UCR (Gormezano, 1972; Mackintosh, 1974).

This anticipatory aspect of the CR is a crucial factor in the adaptive significance of the behavior elicited in classical conditioning experiments. Putting on the hat of a designer of an intelligent problem solver, it would seem desirable to have a mechanism that is able to extract predictive regularities in its input so as to make a representation of a predicted event occur at the earliest time at which that event can be predicted with reasonable certainty. A prediction that is available only at the same time as, or later than the event predicted is no more useful in guiding behavior than no prediction at all; and, assuming a competitive environment, the earlier the prediction is available, the better. Moreover, internal predictive representations might act as predictive cues for other internal events, creating the possibility for effectively "compressing" the time scale in a manner similar to what would happen if we were to tape-record something at one tape speed ("real time") and play it back at a higher speed ("faster than real time"). The utility of predictive methods is well established in engineering applications (Box & Jenkins, 1976), and the adaptive advantage to an organism possessing these capabilities is clear.

The fact that anticipatory CRs are possible at all is problematic for many neural theories. For example, many mathematical interpretations of the Hebbian postulate require simultaneous pairing of the UCS and CS signals at the adaptive element, thus implying an optimal ISI of zero. Because the dependency of conditioning on the ISI is generally recognized, delays in the CS pathway are often suggested to bring the behavior closer to animal data (Burke, 1966; Uttley, 1979). Such delays can be used to reproduce the experimental observation that the CS onset must precede the UCS onset in order for conditioning to occur, but they do not by themselves explain the experimental observation that the CR onset generally also occurs before the UCS onset. Such delays necessarily delay CR onset at least until the time of UCS onset, thereby preventing the CR latency from ever being shorter than the ISI required for conditioning. Reverberatory trace mechanisms in the CR pathway are more satisfactory, but they do not allow for precise temporal localization of the CS.

Let us examine the behavior of the aforementioned adaptive element for a special case of classical conditioning in which the CS and the UCS are rectangular pulses, the CS associative strength is initially zero, and the trace $\bar{s}$ takes the form $\bar{s}(t) = s(t - 1)$. Figure 7.3a shows the adaptive element analog of

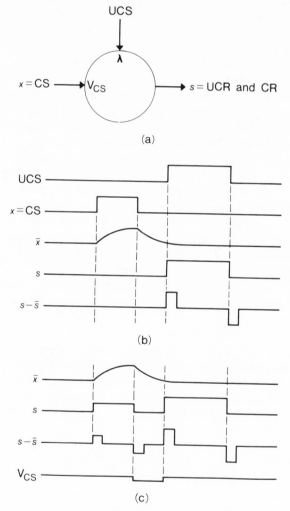

FIG. 7.3 Analog of classical conditioning with a single CS. (a) The adaptive element configuration. (b) Time courses of the model variables for the first trial. (c) Time courses of the model variables after complete conditioning. Note that the element response (s) to the CS anticipates the UCS. (Reprinted from Barto & Sutton, 1982).

this situation, and Figs. 7.3b and 7.3c show the signal time courses we now describe. On the first trial, the occurrence of the CS causes an increase in the eligibility $\bar{x}$ of the CS pathway that persists for some time after CS offset. When the UCS occurs, it causes a positive change in s at its onset and an equal but negative change at its offset. Because eligibility $\bar{x}$ is greater at the time of UCS onset than at the time of UCS offset, V_{CS} is caused to have a net increase: It increases at UCS onset and decreases by a lesser amount at UCS offset (Fig. 7.3b).

On the second trial, V_{CS} is no longer zero so that CS occurrence causes changes in s in addition to those caused by UCS occurrence (Fig. 7.3c). The increase in s at CS onset has no effect on V_{CS} because eligibility is zero (we are assuming that the intertrial interval is long enough to let eligibility decay to zero between trials). The decrease in s at CS offset, however, occurs during high eligibility and therefore causes a decrease in V_{CS}. The UCS causes an increase in V_{CS} as on the first trial, but the net result of both the CS and UCS is less of an increase than on Trial 1. With additional trials, V_{CS} increases until the positive effect of the UCS is counterbalanced by the negative effect of the CS offset. The process therefore stabilizes in the sense that eventually V_{CS} will experience no net change per trial (although it will in general continue to change during these trials). Stability is achieved through negative feedback due to increases in V_{CS} causing increased decreases in V_{CS} at CS offset. Figure 7.4, Trials 0–10, shows a typical acquisition curve plotting the associative strength after each trial[1].

Fig. 7.3c shows that the value of s shows a response to the CS and the UCS. The later response is assumed to contribute to the UCR whereas the earlier one is assumed to contribute to the CR. Thus, the CR component anticipates the UCS onset and the UCR onset. Here, the CR latency is zero because we have assumed that there is no delay in the input/output response of the element, but the ISI must be positive for conditioning to occur. The basis for this anticipatory behavior is clearly the prolonged eligibility trace. If an event regularly precedes another event by an amount of time spannable by this trace's duration, then the association between these events can be "recorded," in a sense, by the adaptive element and "played back" at a much faster time scale.

The adaptive element is also capable of doing something more subtle than this. Because activity on any input pathway with nonzero weight causes changes in s, this activity can cause changes in the weights of other pathways. Thus, a previously conditioned CS can act as a UCS for a second CS. This also can occur in a Hebbian element analog of classical conditioning, but

---

[1]This acquisition curve is strictly negatively accelerated whereas experimental acquisition curves generally have an initial period of positive acceleration. Extensions of models similar to our adaptive element have been proposed to remedy this (Frey & Sears, 1978).

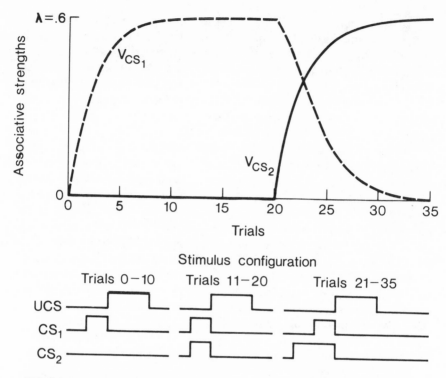

FIG. 7.4 Analog of a blocking experiment. Trials 0–10: Acquisition curve for a single CS in Part I of the blocking experiment. Trials 11–20: Part II of the blocking experiment. CS_1 and CS_2 are identically paired; the formation of an association from CS_2 is blocked due to prior conditioning to CS_1. Trials 21–35: Interaction of stimulus context and anticipatory effects. Blocking is reversed because CS_2 is an earlier predictor of UCS occurrence. (Reprinted from Barto & Sutton, 1982).

when coupled to the anticipatory capabilities of our element, some novel consequences appear. Figure 7.5 shows a simulated experimental arrangement in which each trial consists of a temporal sequence of four CSs (i.e., a serial compound CS) followed by a UCS. Only the CS that occurs immediately before the UCS (i.e., CS_1) initiates an eligibility trace that reaches far enough into the future to permit conditioning to occur. At first, then, only the associative strength of CS_1 increases. As an association from CS_1 is forming, however, CS_1 occurrence causes changes in s and thereby acts as a UCS for the preceding CS, that is, for CS_2. In turn, CS_2 acts as a UCS for CS_3, etc. Figure 7.5 shows the acquisition curves of this higher-order conditioning process. During this process, the CR onset moves back in time from the time of CS_1 onset to the earlier time of CS_4 onset. Kehoe, Gibbs, Garcia, and Gormezano (1979) observed a strong effect of this nature for rabbit nictating-membrane response (see also Gormezano & Kehoe, in press). Chaining of associations in this manner (by a single element) permits conditioning to occur for ISIs much longer than those that can be spanned by a single eligibility trace, provided there are regularly occurring intervening events. Under such conditions, the anticipatory CR will tend to begin at the earliest time at which the UCS can be predicted with reasonable certainty irrespective of the eligibility trace duration. We discuss the significance of this capability from a problem-solving perspective in more detail in a later section ("Assignment of Credit").

Stimulus Context Effects and Orthogonalization

In classical conditioning experiments the associative strength of the stimuli that act as context for a CS on a trial can nullify or even reverse the effect of the occurrence of the UCS on that trial. In this section, we discuss two examples of stimulus context effects, known as *blocking* and *conditioned inhibition,* and show how the adaptive element already described is able to produce these effects. We then explain this by relating our element to the Rescorla–Wagner model of classical conditioning and discuss the significance of this behavior from a problem-solving point of view. In particular, we observe that the stimulus context effects that animals exhibit can be inter-

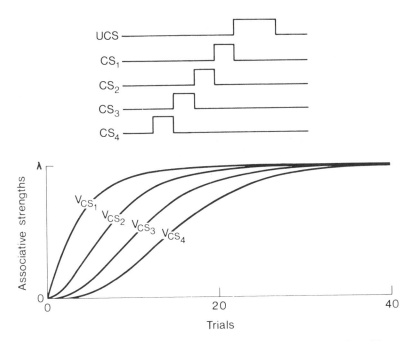

FIG. 7.5   Serially compound CSs. As their associative strengths increase, later CSs serve as UCSs for earlier CSs. (Reprinted from Barto & Sutton, 1982).

preted as the result of a process that "orthogonalizes" stimulus vectors, a process of considerable practical importance.

A typical blocking experiment consists of two parts. In Part I, one stimulus, CS_1, is paired with the UCS at an appropriate ISI until the associative strength between CS_1 and the UCS reaches its asymptotic value. In Part II, CS_1 continues to be paired with the UCS, but another stimulus, CS_2, co-occurs with CS_1. Although CS_2 is appropriately paired with the UCS in Part II, it conditions very poorly, if at all, compared to a control group lacking prior Part I conditioning to CS_1 (see, for example, Hilgard & Bower, 1975). The results of a simulation of blocking using our adaptive element are illustrated in Trials 0–20 of Fig. 7.4. For the first 10 trials, CS_1 was presented alone and followed by the UCS, and for Trials 11–20, CS_2 was presented identically paired with CS_1, and both were followed by the UCS. During trials 11–20, changes in V_{CS_2} were blocked because s did not change while the CS_2 pathway was eligible.

Conditioned inhibition is another stimulus context effect involving at least two CSs, denoted $CS+$ and $CS-$. Suppose the occurrence of $CS+$ alone is always followed by the UCS, but the co-occurrence of $CS+$ and $CS-$ is never followed by the UCS. For this paradigm, the associative strength V_{CS+} increases so that $CS+$ produces a CR, but V_{CS-} becomes negative so that a CR does not follow the co-occurrence of $CS+$ and $CS-$; $CS-$ becomes a conditioned inhibitor of the CR. Figure 7.6 shows the results of a simulation of this procedure using our adaptive element.

Perhaps the best way to explain how our adaptive element produces these effects is to relate it to the Rescorla–Wagner model, which was devised to describe these effects in animal behavior (Rescorla & Wagner, 1972). The Rescorla–Wagner model is based on the view that learning occurs only when expectations are violated. According to this view, for example, blocking occurs because Part I training creates an expectation of the UCS that is not disrupted in Part II. When the activity trace $\bar{s}$ in Equation 2 is interpreted as providing the expected value of the actual activity s, then Equation 2 resembles the Rescorla–Wagner model because it implies that eligible pathways are modified whenever the actual value of s differs from the expected value $\bar{s}$. The term $s - \bar{s}$ is a measure of how strongly the current activity confirms or contradicts the previously formed expectation. Sutton and Barto (1981b) discuss the Rescorla–Wagner model and these correspondences in detail. Anticipatory aspects of classical conditioning and ISI dependency are not addressed by the Rescorla–Wagner model because, unlike our element, it is a trial-level model that does not distinguish between different times within each trial.

It is a striking fact that the Rescorla–Wagner model, which was formulated to describe compactly a wide variety of effects observed in animal learning experiments, is identical to an algorithm for iteratively computing the inverse

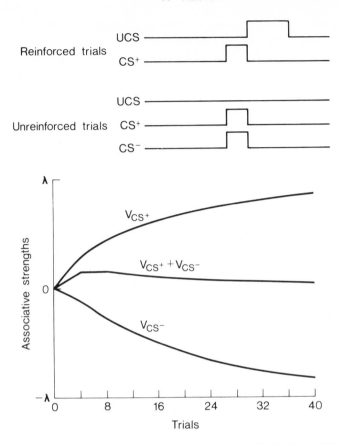

FIG. 7.6   Analog of a conditioned inhibition experiment. CS + is always followed by the UCS, but the co-occurrence of CS + and CS − is never followed by the UCS. CS − becomes a conditioned inhibitor of the CR. (Reprinted from Barto & Sutton, 1982).

of a linear transformation, a process having many practical problem-solving applications. This algorithm has a long history in mathematics and appeared in the form of an adaptive element developed by Widrow and Hoff (1960), which they called an "adaline" (for *ada*ptive *line*ar). Closely related adaptive elements are those used in Rosenblatt's "perceptron" (1962) and Uttley's "informon" (1979). Consider a set $X = \{X^\alpha, 1 \le \alpha \le k\}$ of stimulus patterns $X^\alpha = (x_1^\alpha, \ldots x_n^\alpha)$ and an associated set of real numbers $Z = \{z^\alpha, 1 \le \alpha \le k\}$ where each z^α is the adaline response desired for stimulus pattern X^α. The weights of an adaline change as follows: for $1 \le i \le n$,

$$w_i(t + 1) = w_i(t) + c[z(t) - \sum_{j=1}^{n} w_j(t)x_j(t)]x_i(t)$$

where $z(t) \in Z$ is the reference or "teacher" signal that provides the desired response to input pattern $X(t) = (x_i(t), \ldots, x_n(t)) \in X$, and c is a positive constant. If the set X of input vectors is linearly independent and an adaline is trained by presenting the adaline with sufficient repetitions of the pairs (X^α, z^α), $1 \leq \alpha \leq k$, it will eventually respond with z^α when presented with X^α alone, $1 \leq \alpha \leq k$. In other words, it will form a weight vector $W^* = (w_1^*, \ldots, w_n^*)$ such that

$$[w_1^*, \ldots, w_n^*] \begin{bmatrix} x_1^\alpha \\ \vdots \\ x_n^\alpha \end{bmatrix} = z^\alpha$$

for $1 \leq \alpha \leq k$.

Widrow and Hoff (1960) proposed associative memory networks similar to those discussed by Anderson and Kohonen in this volume but consisting of adalines (although Widrow's work considerably predated this use of the term *associative memory*). Amari (1977a, 1977b) and Kohonen and Oja (1976) discuss similar networks. An associative memory network consisting of adalines does not require orthogonal input, or "key," vectors in order to obtain perfect recall peformance. Amari (1977a, 1977b) calls this "orthogonal learning" because nonorthogonal patterns are "orthogonalized" by the network. Moreover, if the set X is not even linearly independent, the system will form weights so as to minimize the mean square error. The process is, in fact, an algorithm for computing a linear regression or, more technically, for finding the Moore–Penrose pseudoinverse of a linear transformation. Duda and Hart (1973) provide a good overview of this general theory in the context of pattern classification.

Both the stimulus context effects of blocking and conditioned inhibition can be seen as instances of "orthogonalization." For a form of blocking, one has the stimulus vector $X^1 = (1, 0)$ representing the occurrence of CS_1 alone and the vector $X^2 = (1, 1)$ representing the co-occurrence of CS_1 and CS_2. These are clearly linearly independent but not orthogonal. The responses desired are $z^1 = z^2 = \lambda$ (as the UCS, and hence the UCR, occurs on both CS_1 alone and $CS_1 + CS_2$ trials). An adaline will form the weight vector $W^* = (\lambda, 0)$ giving

$$[\lambda, 0] \begin{bmatrix} 1 \\ 0 \end{bmatrix} = [\lambda, 0] \begin{bmatrix} 1 \\ 1 \end{bmatrix} = \lambda$$

Equivalently, the process solves the matrix equation

$$[w_1, w_2] \begin{bmatrix} 1 & 1 \\ 0 & 1 \end{bmatrix} = [\lambda, \lambda]$$

for w_1 and w_2 by effectively finding the inverse of the 2×2 matrix whose columns are the stimulus patterns X^1 and X^2. Blocking appears because w_2 turns out to be zero.

For conditioned inhibition, one has the vectors $X^1 = (1, 0)$ for CS + occurrence and $X^2 = (1, 1)$ for the co-occurrence of CS + and CS − . These are the same linearly independent but nonorthogonal vectors that represent the blocking experiment. The desired responses are $z^1 = \lambda$ and $z^2 = 0$ because the UCS is absent for CS − . An adaline will produce the weight vector $W^* = (\lambda, -\lambda)$, showing that CS + eventually excites the element and CS − eventually inhibits it. Again, the process solves a matrix equation.

These stimulus context effects, and others that we have not discussed, provide evidence that animals "orthogonalize" their stimulus patterns during classical conditioning experiments. We think the independent discovery of this orthogonalization algorithm, in one case to describe animal behavior and in the other case to provide solutions to practical problems, is a remarkable instance of how purely theoretical problem-solving considerations can illuminate the adaptive significance of animal behavior. The adaptive element defined by Equations 1 and 2 orthogonalizes input patterns by virtue of its similarity to an adaline (and hence to the Rescorla–Wagner model) while also preserving some of the anticipatory aspects of classical conditioning. We have not yet thoroughly explored how these two aspects of our element's behavior interact, but an example of this interaction is provided by the results shown in Fig. 7.4, Trials 21–35. Here blocking is reversed because CS_2 begins earlier than a previously conditioned CS_1, suggesting that stimulus context effects occur insofar as they are consistent with the tendency to extract the earliest predictors of the UCS. We know of no attempts to perform this experiment on an animal preparation.

We have also not yet thoroughly explored the possibilities suggested by the use of our classical conditioning element in the associative memory paradigm discussed by Anderson and Kohonen in this volume. In one study, however, we used these elements to form a predictive associative memory that served as an internal model to evaluate proposed, but not overtly executed actions (Sutton & Barto, 1981a; see Fig. 7.7). We illustrated how this configuration was able to account for some of the difficult features of an experiment demonstrating "latent learning" in animals. We now focus on another type of adaptive element that was used in the "action selector" component shown in Fig. 7.7.

GOAL–SEEKING ADAPTIVE ELEMENTS

The adaptive element described in the preceding section operates in a completely open-loop mode: Its operation does not depend in any way on its being able to influence its input signals, as is appropriate because the classical conditioning paradigm was designed to prevent response contingencies (although in practice it may be impossible to remove all such contingencies). Instrumental (cued operant) conditioning, on the other hand, is learning that

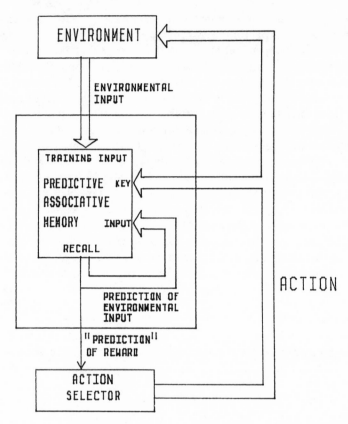

FIG. 7.7   The use of a predictive associative memory as an internal model enabling proposed actions to be evaluated before they are executed. (Reprinted from Sutton & Barto,
1981a).

occurs in experimental paradigms that do involve response contingencies.
Reinforcement may be given or withheld depending on the animal's response.
If a system can exert such control over its input, it is possible to speak of goal-
seeking behavior in which, for example, the system acts so as to obtain appe-
titive stimuli and avoid aversive stimuli. Despite common belief to the contrary, nontrivial forms of response-contingent learning have received very
little attention from adaptive network theorists[2]. Recognizing this, Klopf
(1972, 1982) proposed that neurons may operate as analogs of instrumental

_____

[2]This may seem a surprising comment, and an adequate defense of it is beyond the scope of the
present chapter. Although the "error-correction" methods employed by the adaline or perception, for example, are often considered to be analogous to "trial-and-error" learning, they are
not. These methods search in the space of weight vectors but not in the space of possible actions.
In Barto and Sutton (1981b) we discuss this in more detail.

conditioning rather than classical conditioning and suggested how this may be accomplished. What follows is a discussion of some of our studies of networks of such goal-seeking components.

The psychological literature on instrumental conditioning and on the relationship between instrumental and classical conditioning is extremely complex. Rather than attempting to carefully integrate our studies of closed-loop learning rules with this literature, as we attempted to do for the open-loop case of classical conditioning, we have instead concentrated on the problem-solving potential of such rules. Here we describe some simulation experiments intended to illustrate these capabilities in a vivid and intuitively satisfying manner. This adaptive element was presented by Barto, Sutton, and Brouwer (1981) and the experiments described here were presented by Barto and Sutton (1981b).

This adaptive element has n input pathways x_i, $1 \leq i \leq n$, a specialized "payoff" pathway z, and an output pathway y. We let $x_i(t)$, $1 \leq i \leq n$, $z(t)$, and $y(t)$ respectively denote the activity on these pathways at time t. As usual, a variable weight with value $w_i(t)$ at time t is associated with each pathway x_i, $1 \leq i \leq n$. Let

$$s(t) = \sum_{i=1}^{n} w_i(t)x_i(t).$$

The output of the element at time t is

$$y(t) = \begin{cases} 1 \text{ if } s(t) + \text{NOISE}(t) > 0 \\ 0 \text{ else} \end{cases} \tag{3}$$

where $\text{NOISE}(t)$ is a normally distributed random variable with mean zero. The weights change according to the following equation:

$$w_i(t) = w_i(t-1) + c[z(t) - z(t-1)]y(t-1)x_i(t-1) \tag{4}$$

for $1 \leq i \leq n$, where c is a positive constant determining the rate of learning.

This adaptive element *searches* for the action that will lead to the largest payoff obtainable in the situations signaled by its stimulus patterns. Suppose the payoff provided to the element at time t is a function of the element's action at time $t-1$ and the stimulus pattern $X(t-1) = (x_1(t-1), \ldots, x_n(t-1))$ present at time $t-1$; that is $z(t) - f[y(t-1), X(t-1)]$. The element is to learn to perform the action $y(t-1)$ in response to the pattern $X(t-1)$ that maximizes $z(t)$. The element searches for this action by trying its various responses to each pattern and settling on the one that turns out to be best. The element need never be directly instructed as to which response is best for each pattern. If the consequences of an action are not returned to the element in one time step as we have assumed here, it is appropriate to replace the terms $z(t-1)$, $y(t-1)$, and $x_i(t-1)$ in Equation 4 with prolonged traces of these signals such as those used in the classical conditioning element described in the previous section.

The random component in the element's response (Equation 3) is essential to this process. Responses are made randomly but are biased in one direction or the other by the sum s. Because s depends on the input patterns through the weights, the weights determine how this probabilistic bias conditionally depends on each input pattern. According to Equation 4, if the element "fired" at $t - 1$ (i.e., $y(t - 1) = 1$) in the presence of nonzero input activity on pathway i (i.e., $x_i(t - 1) > 0$), perhaps due to an excitatory effect of signal x_i or perhaps by chance, *and* this was followed by an increase in payoff (i.e., $z(t) - z(t - 1) > 0$), then firing in the presence of signal x_i is made more likely by incrementing weight w_i. Similarly, the firing probability is decreased if the payoff decreases. The noise in the response, then, is essential to the learning process because it generates trials in the absence of any preestablished influence from sensory input and continues to generate trials as this influence is established. Conducting a search in this probabilistic manner also permits the element to improve its performance (in terms of the amount of payoff received) even if the environment provides payoff in a nondeterministic manner, a property whose importance will become more clear when we consider a network of these elements.

Hill Climbing and Chemotaxis

The adaptive element just described implements an elaboration of a goal-seeking strategy that occurs in certain simple organisms. Fraenkel and Gunn (1961) discuss a number of methods used by animals for finding and remaining near light or dark areas, warm or cool areas, or, in general, for approaching attractants and avoiding repellents. One of the most primitive mechanisms is a strategy that they called klinokinesis, the most intensely studied example of which occurs in the behavior of various types of bacteria such as *Escherichia coli, Salmonella typhimurium,* or *Bacillus subtilis.* This manifestation of klinokinesis, known as bacterial chemotaxis, was discovered in the 1880s and was recently reviewed by Koshland (1979). These bacteria propel themselves along relatively straight paths by rotating (!) flagella. With what at first appears to be a random frequency, they reverse flagellar rotation, which causes a momentary disorganization of the flagellar filaments. This causes the bacterium to stop and tumble in place. As the disorganized flagellum continues to rotate in the new direction, its filaments twist together again, causing the bacterium to move off in some random new direction. If the attractant is getting stronger, the probability of reversing flagellar rotation decreases, thereby increasing the probability that the bacterium will continue to move in the same direction; whereas if the attractant level drops, the probability increases that the bacterium's flagellum will reverse and cause the bacterium to swim off in a randomly chosen new direction. Runs in directions leading up the attractant gradient therefore tend to be longer than runs in directions leading down the gradient. As a result of this strategy, bacteria are able to find and remain in the vicinity of the peaks of attractant distributions. Selfridge (1978) points out the general utility of this basic mechanism, which he calls "run-and-twiddle"—if things are getting better, keep doing whatever you are doing; if things are getting worse, do something (anything!) else. It is a very effective strategy, particularly when gradient information is very noisy.

To see how the adaptive element defined by Equations 3 and 4 implements an analog of this procedure, consider an element that receives only a single input signal, say x_0, in addition to the payoff, and assume that x_0 has a constant value of 1, that is, $x_0(t) = 1$ for all t. The weight w_0 associated with this signal changes according to Equation 4, where the term $x_i(t - 1) = 1$ for all t. The payoff level $z(t)$ represents the level of attractant sensed by the element at time t. Thus, if "firing" is followed by an increase in attractant level, then firing is made more likely. Note that we can consider the single constant input and its weight as a convenient means of specifying a variable threshold (so that the constant input need not really be supplied from the element's environment). If upper and lower bounds were imposed on the value of w_0 and if the learning constant c were large enough, then a single "move" up or down the attractant gradient would respectively cause the element to "continue doing what it was doing" or to "do something else" (with a high probability).

Rather than directly simulating a spatial version of "running" and "twiddling" using a single element, we simulated an "organism" whose locomotion is controlled by four adaptive elements, each controlling movement in one of the four cardinal directions; it moves north if Element 1 fires, south if Element 2 fires, etc. In case two elements fire simultaneously, then an appropriate compound move is made, for example, northwest. A sort of "reciprocal inhibition" is used to reduce the probability that the north and south or the east and west elements fire together. We assume that each move is a fixed distance and is completed in a single time step. Clearly, we were not attempting to model in any detailed manner the motor control system of an actual organism, and we have not optimized this hill-climbing strategy. Figure 7.8 shows the simulated organism's trail in an environment containing a "tree" as the center of an attractant distribution that decreases linearly with distance from the tree. The organism (shown as an asterisk) approaches the tree and remains in its vicinity.

Associative Search

The simulated organism climbing the attractant distribution in Fig. 7.8 is not forming long-term memory traces. If we were to move it back to its starting

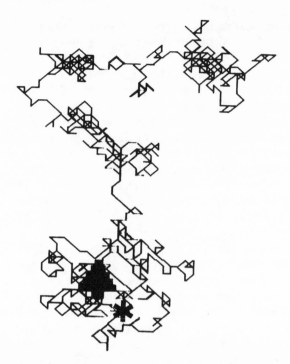

FIG. 7.8   Chemotacticlike behavior of a network of goal-seeking adaptive elements. The "organism," shown as an asterisk, started in the upper right and generated the trail shown as it climbed an attractant distribution whose peak is marked by the location of the "tree." (Reprinted from Barto & Sutton, 1981b).

position, it would take just as long (on the average) to move toward the tree; nothing was learned during the first excursion. This suggests that the other input pathways to the elements controlling locomotion might provide information that can be used to guide the hill-climbing procedure and that their weights might provide useful long-term memory traces. The following simulation experiments were designed to explore the coupling of associative learning capabilities with chemotacticlike behavior. To the spatial environment already described, we added four "landmarks," each of which emits a distinctive "odor" that decays with distance from the landmark (Fig. 7.9a). These odors are neutral in the sense that they are not attractants or repellents but can serve as cues as to location in space.

Figure 7.9b shows the network of four adaptive elements that controls movement in the manner described. These input pathways are labeled vertically on the left according to the landmarks to which they respond. The location of the organism, then, determines the input pattern it receives. The shaded input pathway N in Fig. 7.9b indicates that the organism is near the north neutral landmark. Given the presence of these other signals, there is no longer a need for the constant input x_0 (although the system still works if it is present). The arrangement of input and output pathways used in Fig. 7.9b permits us to show the connection weights as circles centered on the intersections of input pathways and the vertical output element "dendrites." We show positive weights as hollow circles and negative weights as solid circles. The sizes of the circles indicate the relative magnitudes of the corresponding weights. The uppermost "tree" input is the payoff pathway z, which has no associated weights. This network is an example of what we have called an "associative search network" (Barto et al., 1981). The matrix of weights forms an associative memory, but unlike those discussed by others, it need not be directly told what associations to store. Instead, it stores the successful results of the chemotacticlike search. With sufficient experience, the system can learn to respond to the configuration of signals at each place with the action that is optimal for that place.

Figure 7.10 illustrates the performance of this system. In this case, noise has been added to the attractant level in order to make the hill-climbing task more difficult. Figure 7.10a shows the trail of an inexperienced organism that starts near the nothern neutral landmark. It eventually remains in the vicinity of the tree. Figure 7.10b shows the trail produced by replacing the organism at its original starting point after it has undergone the experience shown in Fig. 7.10a. It now proceeds directly to the tree, clearly benefiting from its earlier experiences. Figure 7.11a shows the network after learning. Nonzero weights have appeared so that, for example, proximity to the northern landmark causes a high probability of movement south because the "odor" of the northern landmark excites the element that causes movement south and inhibits the one that causes movement north. Figure 7.11b shows the results of learning as a vector field in which each vector shows the average direction that the organism will take on its *first* step from any place. The vector field is the organism's map of its environment (it is never literally present in the environment). Moreover, it should be clear that the organism would follow this map even if the tree and its attractant distribution were to be removed (so long as the neutral landmarks remained). Although the problem is simple enough for this network to solve by forming a linear associative mapping, it illustrates how adaptively significant behavior can be achieved naturally by combining associative learning with chemotacticlike strategies. Further discussion of this example is provided in Barto and Sutton (1981b).

Although some accounts of learning in the cybernetic literature essentially equate learning and hill climbing, here we see an example of a hill climber that learns. This is very important from a problem-solving perspective. Search is an essential element of almost any problem-solving task (see, for example, Minsky, 1963), but it is often essential to minimize explicit search in order to gain efficiency. The landmark-guided hill-climbing example illustrates how the results of explicit searches can be transferred to an associative

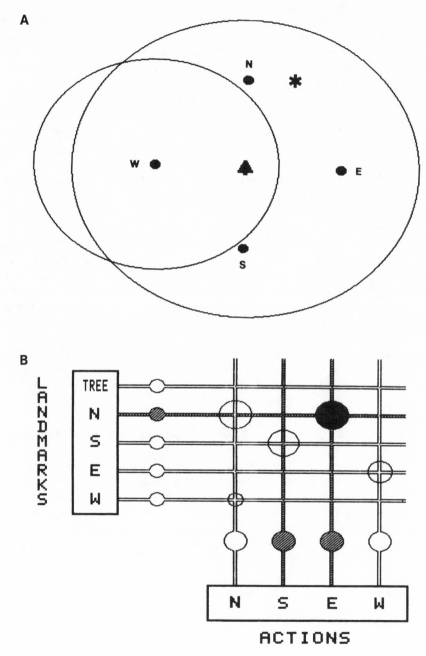

FIG. 7.9

A   B

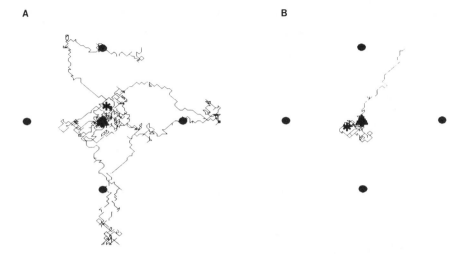

FIG. 7.10   Chemotacticlike behavior combined with associative learning. (a) The trail of an inexperienced organism that starts near the northern neutral landmark. Hill climbing is difficult because noise has been added to the attractant level, but the organism eventually remains in the vicinity of the attractant peak. (b) The trail produced by an experienced organism. After the experience shown in (a), the organism is placed in its original starting position. It now proceeds directly to the tree, clearly benefiting from its previous experience.

long-term store so that in future encounters with similar (but not necessarily identical) situations the system need only access the store in order to find out what to do. The associative search network shows how all of this can be accomplished without centralized control. It is thus an improvement over a nonlearning search method while also offering an improvement over the usual storage methods for associative memories because the optimal responses need not be known a priori by the environment, the system, or the

FIG. 7.9   *(Opposite page)* (a) A spatial environment in which the attracting "tree" is surrounded by four other landmarks. The landmarks each possess a distinctive "odor" that can be sensed at a distance but that is not an attractant. Odor distributions decrease linearly from their associated landmarks and become undetectable at a certain distance (indicated for landmark '*W*' by the surrounding circle). (b) A network of goal-seeking adaptive elements. The five input pathways are labeled vertically on the left according to the landmarks to which they respond. The shaded input pathway *N* indicates that the organism is near the north neutral landmark. The four output pathways controlling actions are labeled horizontally at the bottom according to the direction of movement they cause. The shaded output elements indicate that a southeast movement is being made. The associative matrix weights are displayed as circles centered on the intersections of the horizontal input pathways and vertical output pathways. Positive weights are shown as hollow circles, and negative weights are shown as solid circles. (Reprinted from Barto & Sutton, 1981b).

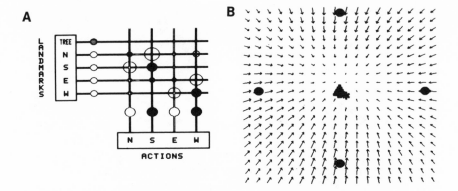

FIG. 7.11 Associative memory contents after learning. (a) The network showing the weights. Nonzero weights have appeared so that, for example, proximity to the northern landmark causes a high probability of moving south because the "odor" of the northern landmark excites action S and inhibits action N. (b) A vector field representation of the associative memory's contents. Each vector shows the most likely direction that the organism will move on its *first* step from any place. Note the generalization to places it has never visited. (Reprinted from Barto & Sutton, 1981b).

system's designer. Future research will focus on networks that combine associative learning with search strategies that are more sophisticated than simple hill climbing.

Neural Signaling and Bacterial Chemotaxis

Koshland (1979) suggests that study of the numerous commonalities between bacterial chemotaxis and other forms of adaptive behavior in single-celled organisms, and the signaling systems of neurons may provide insight into neural mechanisms. Like bacteria, neurons possess receptors that detect chemical signals from their environments. A bacterium's sensory-processing system produces signals that control its motor response by altering the probability of flagellar reversal. Neurons similarly respond to chemically mediated afferent signals and produce action potentials as "motor" responses. Koshland (1979) hypothesizes that many features of bacterial chemotaxis can be accounted for by a model in which random variations in the concentration of a hypothetical tumble regulator substance X are modulated by changes in attractant concentrations. Flagellar reversal occurs whenever the concentration of X exceeds a threshold. Suppose X is formed at rate V_f and decomposed at rate V_d. If an increase in the level of attractant sensed causes a fast increase in V_f and a slower increase in V_d, then the intracellular concentration of X will show a transient increase to any sustained increase in attractant level, and a transient decrease to any sustained decrease (Fig. 7.12), thus causing the appropriate hill-climbing behavior. This is the same sort of "differentiation" accomplished by the term $s(t) - \bar{s}(t)$ of the classical conditioning element (Equation 2) and the term $z(t) - z(t - 1)$ of the goal-seeking element (Equation 4). More specifically, the value of the term $s(t) + \text{NOISE}(t)$ in Equation 3 functionally corresponds to the concentration of the hypothetical substance X in Koshland's model. Mechanisms similar to those suggested by Koshland for bacterial chemotaxis could provide a basis for neurons to exhibit related behavior.

It is an intriguing hypothesis that neurons implement goal-seeking strategies related to those of single-celled organisms. Perhaps it will prove useful to view neurons as swimming (in a metaphorical sense, of course) in an environment of contingencies determined by the nervous system of which they are a part and the organism and its environment to whose survival they contribute. Important aspects of a neuron's behavior may involve its ability to influence its own input when operating in its usual environment. This influence may extend through the environment external to the entire organism, as well as through local internal feedback loops. In order to experimentally investigate this hypothesis, single neurons would need to be studied in closed-loop control situations in which their efferent activity could influence, perhaps after considerable delay, their afferent activity according to experimentally known and controllable transformations.

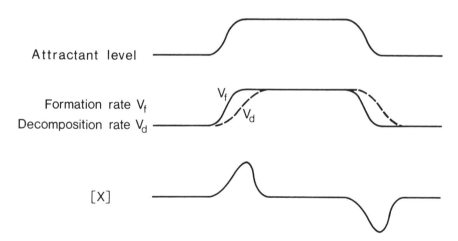

FIG. 7.12   Hypothetical mechanism for detecting attractant gradient in bacterial chemotaxis (from Koshland, 1979). The formation and decomposition rates V_f and V_d of a hypothetical substance X are influenced by the attractant level. Both V_f and V_d follow the attractant level sensed, but V_d changes more slowly than V_f. This results in the concentration of X responding to changes in attractant levels. (After Barto & Sutton, 1981c).

ASSIGNMENT OF CREDIT

We have described two types of adaptive elements that share many basic features but whose behaviors have a different character, one closely related to classical conditioning, and the other related to instrumental conditioning and bacterial chemotaxis. We have argued that both types of behavior would confer adaptive advantages to any organism possessing them, but we have not suggested how these forms of behavior might be related. Here, we propose that this relationship can be understood in terms of what has been called the "assignment of credit problem." Suppose success is achieved by a complex mechanism after operating over a considerable period of time (for example, a chess-playing program wins a game). To what particular decisions made by what particular components should the successs be attributed? And, if failure results, what decisions deserve blame? The magnitude of this problem is most forcefully appreciated by those actually attempting to construct systems capable of learning to improve performance in complex tasks. This is closely related to the problem known as the "mesa" or "plateau" problem (Minsky, 1963; Minsky & Selfridge, 1960). The performance evaluation function available to a learning system may consist of large level regions in which hill-climbing degenerates to exhaustive search. Only a few of the situations obtainable by the learning system and its environment are known to be desirable, and these situations may occur rarely.

An approach to one aspect of this problem is illustrated by the network of goal-seeking components described previously. At each time step, each element produces a component of a total output pattern. If a pattern produces an increase in the performance evaluation (i.e., if the organism moves up the attractant gradient), to what element or elements should success be attributed? The network solves this problem by assigning credit to *any* element that happened to fire, whether or not its firing was actually causal in producing success. The probabilistic nature of the search procedure, however, allows any misleading consequences of this strategy to be averaged out with repeated trials (and we are reminded of the philosophical problem of truly distinguishing causality from correlation). More technically, part of each element's operation implements what is known as a stochastic learning automaton optimization method (see, for example, Narendra & Thathachar, 1974) and is capable of improving its performance under the uncertainty produced by the unknown and random influences of the other elements on its own payoff. Of course, the larger the network, the more trials will be required in general for credit to be apportioned correctly. Thus, this method alone will not suffice for large networks. Another part of the solution may be to permit interconnections to form between elements and to effectively assign credit to linked assemblies of elements rather than to individual elements.

Our experiments with layered networks of goal-seeking elements suggest that this approach indeed works, but a complete discussion is beyond the scope of the present chapter.

Another aspect of the assignment of credit problem concerns temporal factors. The utility of making a certain action may depend on the sequence of actions of which it is a part, and an indication of improved performance may not occur until the entire sequence has been completed. The landmark learning task presented here does not illustrate this problem because we assumed that an action was always evaluated in a single time step. An approach to this problem has been discussed by Minsky (1963) and has been used successfully in Samuel's (1959) famous learning checkers-playing program. The idea is to interpret predictions of future reward as rewarding events themselves. In other words, neutral stimulus events can themselves become reinforcing if they regularly occur before events that are intrinsically reinforcing. This phenomenon is observed in animal learning experiments in which neutral stimuli can become "secondary reinforcers" if they predict "primary reinforcement." This has two consequences. First, a prediction of eventual reward can reinforce the actions that precede that prediction, thereby eliminating the delay in obtaining useful evaluative feedback. Second, a prediction of reward can provide reinforcement to the learning process by which the predictions themselves are formed, permitting the formation, via associative transfer, of predictions of predictions, etc. This is, in fact, the mechanism employed by the classical conditioning element described in the second section of this chapter. Its anticipatory behavior, coupled with its ability to produce higher-order conditioning, is ideally suited for providing evaluative information to a goal-seeking system that is more useful than information directly available from its environment. This view parallels the CR-mediational theories of instrumental conditioning proposed by animal learning theorists (Gormezano & Kehoe, in press). Moreover, the classical conditioning element turns out to implement an algorithm remarkably similar to a part of the actual algorithm used by Samuel in his checkers-playing program. We are currently investigating systems that combine both types of adaptive elements and that face control tasks characterized by variably delayed reinforcement, and it may be possible to devise a single relatively simple element that combines both types of behavior.

CONCLUSION

In this article, we have described some of the results of a research program intended to reexamine the potential for networks of neuronlike adaptive elements to provide a computational substrate for solving nontrivial problems.

We have highlighted examples of how adaptively significant features of animal behavior and pure problem-solving considerations converge: the anticipatory nature of classical conditioning and the necessity to construct internal evaluation criteria to solve problems involving variably delayed reinforcement; stimulus context effects of classical conditioning and the utility of orthogonalizing stimulus patterns for associative storage; bacterial chemotaxis and the necessity of search in problem solving. We have described an adaptive element that preserves some of these features of classical conditioning and an element that combines the goal-seeking nature of chemotaxis with associative learning. Networks of the latter type of element conduct searches, store the results of these searches, and access these results to aid future searches. They also eliminate the necessity for the learning system's environment to know the optimal associations. Further, this is accomplished without centralized control. Our present research is directed toward extending these capabilities in order to produce networks that are able to solve problems that have proved resistant to standard problem-solving methods.

ACKNOWLEDGMENTS

This research was supported by the Air Force Office of Scientific Research and the Avionics Laboratory (Air Force Wright Aeronautical Laboratories) through contracts F33615-77-C-1191 and F33615-80-C-1088. The authors wish to thank M. A. Arbib, W. L. Kilmer, D. N. Spinelli, A. H. Klopf, J. W. Moore, and O. G. Selfridge for their many valuable criticisms and contributions.

REFERENCES

Amari, S. A mathematical approach to neural systems. In J. Metzler (Ed.), *Systems neuroscience.* New York: Academic Press, 1977. (a)

Amari, S. Neural theory of association and concept-formation. *Biol. Cybernetics,* 1977, *26,* 175–185. (b)

Arbib, M. A. *The metaphorical brain.* New York: Wiley–Interscience, 1972.

Barto, A. G., & Sutton, R. S. *Goal-seeking components for adaptive intelligence: An initial assessment.* Technical Report. Avionics Laboratory, Air Force Wright Aeronautical Laboratories, Wright–Patterson Air Force Base, Ohio, 1981. (a)

Barto, A. G., & Sutton, R. S. Landmark learning: An illustration of associative search. *Biol. Cybernetics,* 1981, *42,* 1–8. (b)

Barto, A. G., & Sutton, R. S. Simulation of anticipatory responses in classical conditioning by a neuron-like adaptive element. *Behavioral Brain Research,* 1982, *4,* 221–235. (c)

Barto, A. G., Sutton, R. S., & Brouwer, P. Associative search network: A reinforcement learning associative memory. *Biol. Cybernetics,* 1981, *40,* 201–211.

Box, G., & Jenkins, G. *Time series analysis: Forecasting and control.* San Francisco: Holden Day, 1976.

Burke, W. Neuronal models for conditioned reflexes. *Nature,* 1966, *210,* 269–271.

Duda, R. O., & Hart, P. E. *Pattern classification and scene analysis.* New York: Wiley, 1973.

Fraenkel, G. S., & Gunn, D. L. *The orientation of animals: Kineses, taxes and compass reactions.* New York: Dover, 1961.

Frey, P. W., & Sears, R. J. Model of conditioning incorporating the Rescorla–Wagner associative axiom, a dynamic attention process, and a catastrophe rule. *Psychol. Rev.,* 1978, *85,* 321–340.

Gormezano, I. Investigations of defense and reward conditioning in the rabbit. In A. H. Black & W. F. Prokasy (Eds.), *Current research and theory.* New York: Appleton–Century–Crofts, 1972.

Gormezano, I., & Kehoe, E. J. Associative transfer in classical conditioning to serial compounds. In M. L. Commons, R. J. Herrnstein, & A. R. Wagner (Eds.), *Quantitative analysis of behavior. Vol. 3: Acquisition.* Cambridge: Ballinger, in press.

Hebb, D. O. *The organization of behavior.* New York: Wiley, 1949.

Hilgard, E. R., & Bower, G. H. *Theories of learning* (4th ed.). Englewood Cliffs, N.J.: Prentice-Hall, 1975.

Kehoe, J. E., Gibbs, C. M., Garcia, E., & Gormezano, I. Associative transfer and stimulus selection in classical conditioning of the rabbit's nictitating membrane response to serial compound CSs. *Journal of Experimental Psychology: Animal Behavior Processes,* 1979, *5,* 1–18.

Kimmell, H. D. Instrumental inhibitory factors in classical conditioning: In W. F. Prokasy (Ed.), *Classical conditioning.* New York: Appleton–Century–Crofts, 1965.

Klopf, A. H. *Brain function and adaptive systems—A heterostatic theory.* Air Force Cambridge Research Laboratories Research Report AFCRL–72–0164, Bedford, Mass., 1972. (A summary appears in Proc. Int. Conf. Syst., Man., Cybern., IEEE Syst., Man, Cybern., Soc., Dallas, Texas, 1974)

Klopf, A. H. Goal-seeking systems from goal-seeking components: Implications for AI. The *Cognition & Brain Theory Newsletter,* 1979, *3,* 2.

Klopf, A. H. *The hedonistic neuron: A theory of memory, learning and intelligence.* Washington, D.C.: Hemisphere Publishing Corp., 1982.

Kohonen, T., & Oja, E. Fast adaptive formation of orthogonalizing filters and associative memory in recurrent networks of neuron-like elements. *Biol. Cybernetics,* 1979, *21,* 85–95.

Koshland, D. E. Jr. A model regulatory system: Bacterial chemotaxis. *Physiol. Rev.,* 1979, *59,* 811–862.

Mackintosh, N. J. *The psychology of animal learning.* New York: Academic Press, 1974.

Mendel, J. M., & McLaren, R. W. Reinforcement-learning control and pattern recognition systems. In J. M. Mendel, & K. S. Fu (Eds.), *Adaptive, learning, and pattern recognition systems: Theory and applications.* New York: Academic Press, 1970.

Minsky, M. L. Steps toward artificial intelligence. In E. A. Feigenbaum, & J. Feldman (Eds.), *Computers and thought.* New York: McGraw-Hill, 1963.

Minsky, M. L., & Selfridge, O. G. Learning in random nets. In C. Cherry (Ed.), *Information theory: Fourth London symposium.* London: Butterworths, 1960.

Narendra, K. S., & Thathachar, M. A. L. Learning automata—a survey. *IEEE Trans. Syst., Man, Cybern.* SMC-4, 1974, *4,* 323–334.

Rescorla, R. A., & Wagner, A. R. A theory of Pavlovian conditioning: Variations in the effectiveness of reinforcement and non-reinforcement. In A. H. Black, & W. F. Prokasy (Eds.), *Classical conditioning II: Current research and theory.* New York: Appleton–Century–Crofts, 1972.

Rosenblatt, F. *Principles of neurodynamics.* New York: Spartan Books, 1962.

Samuel, A. L. Some studies in machine learning using the game of checkers. *IBM J. Res. and Dev.,* 1959, *3,* 210–229.

Selfridge, O. G. *Tracking and trailing: Adaptation in movement strategies.* Unpublished draft, August 1, 1978.

Sutton, R. S., & Barto, A. G. An adaptive network that constructs and uses an internal model of its world. *Cognition & Brain Theory,* 1981, *4,* 217–246. (a)

Sutton, R. S., & Barto, A. G. Toward a modern theory of adaptive networks: Expectation and prediction. *Psychol. Rev.,* 1981, *88,* 135–170. (b)

Uttley, A. M. *Information transmission in the nervous system.* London: Academic Press, 1979.

Widrow, G., & Hoff, M. E. Adaptive switching circuits. In *1960 IRE WESCON Convention Record,* 1960, Part 4, 96–104.

8 What Hebb Synapses Build

James A. Anderson
Brown University

Most of the chapters in this volume arose from a workshop on synaptic modifiability and its implications for brain organization. A major concern of the volume is the biology of synaptic plasticity and explanations of experimental results. This chapter and several others embark on a slightly different way of studying the same question. Instead of asking "How it works?" we ask questions like "Does working that way get you anything?"

In the neurosciences, theory is in very bad repute. Over the past decade, neuroscience has become more and more empirical. Mentioning nervous system models is usually good for a chuckle in a group of experimentalists. This current reaction is in sharp contrast to more remote history. It was considered quite respectable for mathematicians such as Norbert Wiener, Walter Pitts, or John von Neumann to speculate about the brain. Granted, they didn't solve the problem, but a lot of useful ideas emerged as a by-product.

And this is the key to the matter. The brain is like nothing else because by its very nature it performs interesting and significant actions. If we try to understand the nervous system, then it is a reasonable conclusion that we will emerge with principles and theoretical structures that will allow us to construct artificial systems that perform the same kinds of acts that brains do. Note the following: If a model does something of "cognitive" interest, then it very well may not matter whether or not that is how the brain does it.

Because we live in an era of giant thinking machines, there are economic rewards as well as academic fame and glory for the development of systems that perform brainlike actions.

Who Studies Brain Organization?

Three identifiable, often noncommunicating groups study the nervous system.

In one group, we have those who are primarily interested in the structure, function, and organization of the human brain. The ties to biology are very close. Theory, when it exists, must be reasonable in terms of what is known of the anatomy and physiology of the central nervous system. Theory need not exist at all, except at the lowest level; description and recitation of factual material are sufficient to ensure tenure.

In the second group are those who study experimental and mathematical psychology. Psychologists of this kind study the brain as directly as a neuroscientist, though not as obviously. A perfectly valid way of characterizing a system is by studying its input/output relationships. The ties to neuroscience are not direct, though always hoped for. Although the goal is to study the structure of cognition and perception by itself, there is always the tacit belief that a "true" model will turn out to be "physiologically correct" when the facts of the situation are known. My own feeling, for what it is worth, is that this group, as a rule, is much more aware of the work of the first than vice versa.

Although these groups typically reside in different buildings on a college campus—the first in the medical school, possibly in a biology department, the second in a psychology department—they are traditional scientists in the following senses. Most research is done in an academic setting. They are subject to the same standards of conduct and verification as any science. The ultimate aim of work is generally to have theories that can be tested experimentally on animals or humans and that can be falsified and verified by the results.

Let us now expand our perspective. The support for the conference generating the chapters in this book came from the Alfred P. Sloan Foundation. The program involved is not neuroscience or psychology, but "cognitive science." It is still not clear exactly what this means. However, what is quite clear is that another group of players has entered the game, a group that has entered before in other guises and already has contributed a great deal to the study of the brain.

This group, generally involved nowadays with digital computers and artificial intelligence, rather than with the kind of traditional mathematics that concerned Norbert Wiener or John von Neumann, cares primarily about performance. Their approach is to consider the functions that brains perform: learning, memory, understanding language, generating language, seeing objects. After the problem is stated in a very general way, formal systems are proposed to perform the same function. Sometimes these formal systems are inspired by intuitions about psychology, sometimes by intuitions about brain structure, sometimes by nothing other than a hunch that they might work.

I think most of us feel that system designed to perform brainlike functions would benefit from knowing a little about how the brain is built and a little about psychology; however, this is not necessarily so. Many functional systems of great utility have no biological counterpart whatsoever — wheels are good examples.

However, the emphasis on performance strikes me as a very useful boundary condition for those of us who attempt to understand mammalian brain organization. Our models must be well enough formulated to be functional and even potentially useful.

Therefore those of us seriously trying to make models of brain organization must be aware that we are subject to the standards of three different scientific disciplines:

1. Models may be oversimplified but must be "physiological" in that their deviations from reality should not be too extreme.

2. They must be psychologically plausible and should give rise to behavior that is in qualitative agreement with psychological data and principles.

3. They must work, or be well formulated enough to be internally consistent and to show signs of doing as much as they claim they can do and perhaps a bit more.

Here, for the next few pages, I describe an attempt to modeling the nervous system that tries to conform to these principles. Professors Kohonen, Cooper, and Barto, in their contributions, discuss aspects of this particular approach. Their models differ in details, but the overall orientation is similar. Therefore part of this chapter provides a brief, simple introduction to a class of parallel, distributed models.

In a book that is in some ways a companion to this, edited by Geoffrey Hinton and myself and entitled *Parallel Models of Associative Memory* (Anderson & Hinton, 1981), examples of cognitive applications of parallel, distributed models of associative memory are described at some length. This chapter is primarily a review of the material presented at greater length there. Applications of these models to cognition are discussed there and in Anderson (in press).

Real neurons tend to be graded in their activity. That is, instead of being on or off, they respond to stimuli in most, though not all cases as continuous valued voltage-to-frequency converters. There are numerous examples of this; a look at one of the *Handbooks of Sensory Physiology* will give real data. Neurons turn voltage or current into firing frequency much as a relatively simple trannsducer might. There are important nonlinearities, but they are sometimes tractable. A modest degree of linearity coupled with some very simple nonlinearities is often a good first approximation.

We also have a complicated set of concepts that arise when we consider the behavior of not just single neurons, but groups of single neurons. It is important to remember that, in mammals, neurons are members of large sets of neurons, one of many with similar connection patterns. It should be emphasized that different neurons, even in the same group, may do different things. For example, two nearby cells in Area 17 may both respond to lines but with different orientations, therefore they would usually tend to respond to different stimuli.

Single Neuron Selectivity

An important problem involves the question of neuronal selectivity. We look at the physiological data and observe that single neurons respond to only a small number of stimuli, that is, they have considerable selectivity. We could then conjecture that when a neuron is active, it signals extremely precise information about the sensory input.

There are many virtues to this position. Cells *do* something. When a cell fires, something specific and important happens because the cell is "meaningful." This position is held by a number of neurophysiologists, at least in informal discussions.

In psychology this model typically is called the "grandmother cell" or "yellow Volkswagen detector" hypothesis.

Numerous problems arise immediately with this model. How can such extreme selectivity develop? There would have been no value to yellow Volkswagen detectors before 1935. There are powerful learning assumptions concealed. There is another class of objections to the model that arises in other contexts. It is hard to make a system of this kind work in a practical sense. There are too many very strong connections between cells to functional reliably in large systems. Models based on this kind of selectivity face the kind of exponential retrieval catastrophes that are a serious problem for most information retrieval systems of any complexity.

Psychological criticisms also operate. How does this system generalize? Does our yellow Volkswagen detector also respond to chartreuse Volkswagens? How about the green Volkswagen detector? The most reasonable alternative explanation is to assume that there is (say) a "yellow" cell and a "Volkswagen" cell. When they become active together (along with many other cells, such as the "automobile cell," "small car cell," "vehicle cell," and so on) they signal "yellow Volkswagen." Perception no longer corresponds to active single cells, but to *groups* of active single cells. The groups can be much more selective that the single cells that comprise them.

Distribution

Models that have this property—that is, consider the simultaneous activities of single elementary entities—are called *distributed*. It is possible to build models of this type, but they have pronounced and somewhat unfamiliar properties. Complex events are not localized. Specific memories do not occupy specific sites. There is the possibility of resonancelike effects. A single unit is of relatively little importance. Next, I discuss some very simple models of this type.

Parallel, Distributed Models: Association

I discuss first two models that were inspired by neuroscience, that perform functions whose utility is required by psychology, and that, when simulated, suggest something about neuroscience that I found unexpected. I discuss models for *association* and for *feature analysis*. More details can be found in Hinton & Anderson (1981), Anderson and Mozer (1981), Anderson, Silverstein, Ritz, and Jones (1977), and Kohonen (1977).

We assume in our models that what is of importance in the operation of the system are patterns of activity shown by many neurons in a set of neurons. Such activity patterns are denoted as vectors, $\mathbf{f}_1, \mathbf{f}_2, \ldots, \mathbf{f}_k$. Vectors of this type are called *state vectors*. It is possible to develop mathematical structures that let these activity patterns act as fundamental primitive entities. We therefore have moved away from individual neurons, which are component parts of these elementary units. Understanding the lawful behavior of state vectors is the key to developing a theory that is both physiologically reasonable and cognitively interesting.

The psychological aspect of memory that inspires these models is association. Association has been known to be a prominent feature of human memory since Aristotle, and all models of cognition I know of use association in one variant or other as the key operation. Psychological association is not a logical process, but associations are formed because of contiguity, similarity, or other events external to the actual association that is formed. The famous "now-print" signal that actually tells the synapses that now is the time to change is probably a chemical message that we may be starting to understand. (See Pettigrew, this volume).

We must propose a general purpose associative system that conforms to the criteria we discussed ealier; notice that the impetus for making a "general purpose" associator is not from neuroscience but from psychology.

With association as our goal, what mechanisms do we have available at the cellular level to form associations?

Virtually all neuroscientists are convinced that precisely specified changes in synaptic coupling store memory. The chapters elsewhere in this volume give numerous examples of physiological evidence supporting this belief. In general, it is impossible to form new neurons after birth, at least in mammals. Large changes in dendritic branching and formation of new synapses are possible in immature organisms, but are unlikely in adults. Therefore changes in strength of preexisting synapses are the most likely candidate for learning in adults. My favorite candidate for the modifiable structure in adult mammalian neocortex is the dendritic spine. These structures seem to respond to experience in some degree and have electrical properties as well as anatomies that seem highly suitable for modification.

In any case, detailed changes in the coupling between cells seems to be the mechanism. The most common departure point for further development seems to be the suggestion made by Donald Hebb in 1949. Hebb's suggestion was stated as follows:

> When an axon of cell A is near enough to excite a cell B and repeatedly or persistently takes part in firing it, some growth process or metabolic changes take place in one or both cells such that A's efficiency as one of the cells firing B, is increased [p. 62].

This suggestion predicts that cells will tend to become correlated in their discharges, and this kind of synapse is sometimes called a correlational synapse.

Several of the chapters in this volume (Levy, Singer, Cooper) review the evidence for modification equations that are similar to those suggested by Hebb. Obviously, the details are of immense importance and interest. Clearly, also, we now have some physiological evidence that such systems exist in mammalian cortex.

The approach taken here is to derive some very straightforward conclusions that arise if we simply assume that a very simple Hebbian scheme exists. We also briefly describe some simple simulations showing how robust these systems can be, and how resistant they are to damage and to parametric variations.

Let us assume in general that synaptic change is related to the magnitude of both pre- and postsynaptic activity. Then we can immediately show that the system can act as a general purpose associator. As suggested by Hebb, correlational synaptic modification leads to associative structures. Because we know that human cognition is very strongly associative, this is a remarkably interesting result.

A Simple System

Suppose we have two sets of N neurons, alpha and beta, that are completely convergent and divergent, that is, every neuron in alpha projects to every neuron in beta. A neuron j in alpha is connected to neuron i in beta by way of a synapse with strength $A(i, j)$. Our first basic assumption, which we have discussed previously, is that we are primarily interested in the behavior of the set of simultaneous individual neuron activities in a group of neurons. We stress pattern of *individual* neuron activities, because our current knowledge of cortical physiology suggests that cells are highly individualistic. We represent these large patterns as state vectors with independent components. We also assume these components can be positive or negative. This can occur if the relevant physiological variable is considered to be the deviation around a nonzero spontaneous activity level (See Fig. 8.1).

Suppose a pattern of activity, **f**, occurs in alpha. Suppose another pattern of activity, **g**, occurs in beta. Suppose that for some reason we wish to associate these two arbitrary patterns. We assume a detailed synaptic modification rule: To associate pattern **f** in alpha with **g** in beta we need to change the set of synaptic weights according to the product of presynaptic activity at a junction with the activity of the postsynaptic cell. Note that this is information locally available at the junction. If $f(j)$ is the activity of cell j in alpha, and $g(i)$ of cell i in beta, then the change in synaptic strength is given by

$$\Delta A(i, j) = \eta f(j)g(i)$$

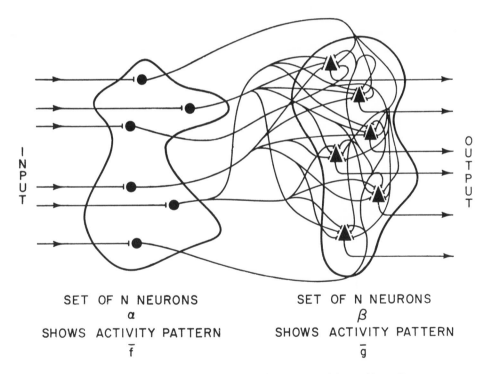

SET OF N NEURONS
α
SHOWS ACTIVITY PATTERN
$\overline{f}$

SET OF N NEURONS
β
SHOWS ACTIVITY PATTERN
$\overline{g}$

FIG. 8.1 We consider the properties of sets of N neurons, alpha, and beta. Every neuron in alpha projects to every neuron in beta. This drawing has $N = 6$ and understates the size and connectivity of the nervous system by several orders of magnitude. (From Anderson, Silverstein, Ritz, & Jones, 1977).

where η is a learning parameter. We see that this defines an n by n matrix $\Delta \mathbf{A}$ of the form $\Delta \mathbf{A} = \eta \mathbf{g} \mathbf{f}^T$. Suppose $\mathbf{f}$ is normalized, so that the inner product $(\mathbf{f}, \mathbf{f}) = 1$, and the learning parameter, η, equals 1. Then, if pattern of activity f recurs in alpha, because beta is connected to alpha, a pattern of activity will also appear in beta. If the activity of a neuron is a simple weighted sum of its inputs as is the *Limulus* eye for example, or as are most simple variants of integrator models for neurons, then we can compute the pattern on beta from the matrix ΔA and from $\mathbf{f}$ as

$$
\begin{aligned}
(\text{pattern on beta}) &= \Delta A f \\
&= g f^T f \\
&= g(f, f) \\
&= g.
\end{aligned}
$$

Suppose that instead of having only one association we have K of them, $(\mathbf{f}_1, \mathbf{g}_1), (\mathbf{f}_2, \mathbf{g}_2), \ldots, (\mathbf{f}_k, \mathbf{g}_k)$, each having associated with an incremental matrix of the form $\Delta \mathbf{A} = \mathbf{g} \mathbf{f}^T$. Because there are only the N synapses in the system, the same synapses must participate in storing all the associations, that is, they are used over and over again. Notice that this is an inexorable consequence of distributed systems and has very powerful consequences. Suppose that the overall connectivity is given by:

$$
\mathbf{A} = \sum_{i=1}^{k} \Delta \mathbf{A}_i
$$

Just as before, what happens when pattern of activity $\mathbf{f}_i$ appears on alpha? Let us do a very simple calculation for the case when the $\mathbf{f}$'s are orthogonal, that is, when the inner product $(\mathbf{f}_i, \mathbf{f}_j) = 0$, if $i \neq j$. (We consider in the next section what happens when we relax this assumption in a related model.)

In the case of orthogonal $\mathbf{f}$'s when $\mathbf{f}_i$ appears on alpha then

$$
\begin{aligned}
(\text{pattern on beta}) &= \mathbf{A} \mathbf{f}_i \\
&= \Delta \mathbf{A}_i \mathbf{f}_i + \sum_{i \neq j} \mathbf{A}_j \mathbf{f}_i \\
&= \mathbf{g}_i + \sum_{i \neq j} \mathbf{g}_j (\mathbf{f}_j \mathbf{f}_i) \\
&= \mathbf{g}_i
\end{aligned}
$$

For orthogonal $\mathbf{f}$'s the system associates random vectors perfectly.

The capacity of the systems is related to N. In the case of association of vectors with orthogonal inputs there is a maximum of N different inputs. Because there are a very large number of neurons in the brain, and even in a single region, this is not as serious a limitation as it might seem. Many of the most powerful generalizing, averaging, and analyzing properties of these models follow from lack of orthogonality at the input.

A Pair of Simulations: Incomplete Connectivity

One desirable feature of a nervous system model should be robustness. Noise, mistakes, unreliable components, and incomplete connectivity should not disastrously degrade the system. From the mathematical structure of the model just presented, we should expect noise resistance, as the operations it uses can often be shown to be optimal in a signal-to-noise sense. Also, there are many averaging operations that should work in our favor.

However, it is easy to check the basic model and variants with a computer simulation to verify its behavior.

We assume for the calculation in the previous section that there was complete connectivity, that is, every presynaptic cell was connected to every postsynaptic cell. This is obviously unrealistic. Let us check what restricting the connectivity does to the system.

We used a 100-dimensional system. Pairs of normalized random vectors were generated and associated according to our learning rule. Elements were generated using a uniform distribution with zero mean. We allowed nonzero matrix elements in different simulations to range from 20% to 100% of the number of elements. The other matrix elements were set to zero; locations were chosen at random. The learning parameter was set so that on the average the output vector would be normalized, that is

$$\eta = \frac{1}{\text{(fraction of nonzero elements)}}.$$

Figure 8.2 shows the results as the number of associated pairs of vectors increases. The cosine of the angle between the actual output of the system, **g** out, and the output presented to and learned by the system, **g**, was computed as a rough measure of goodness of recall. Perfect recall would have a cosine of one.

It can be seen that limited connectivity obviously affects the number of pairs of random vectors that can be associated, but even at 20% connectivity such a memory still serves as a useful associator if the number of stored pairs is small compared to the dimensionality of the system.

Error Correction

The presence of other, nonorthogonal associations obviously leads to inaccurate and noisy recall, particularly if connectivity is incomplete. It would be nice to have some kind of error-correcting procedure to force the system to be accurate if that were desirable. It is easy to modify the basic rule slightly to accomplish this. We assume that learning a particular pair of associations can potentially occur many times, that is, a particular **f** and **g** will appear

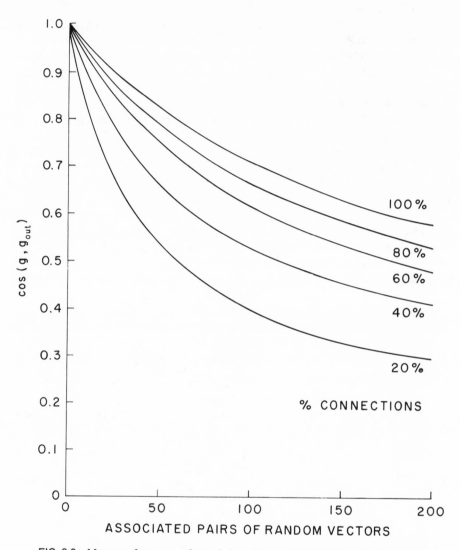

FIG. 8.2 Measure of accuracy of association with a partially filled matrix of synaptic weights. Pairs of 100-dimensional normalized random vectors (uniformly distributed element values with zero mean) were associated according to the simple rule discusssed in the text, but with only randomly chosen 20, 40, 60, 80, or 100% of elements allowed to be nonzero. As a measure of retrieval accuracy, the cosine of the angle between the correct (i.e., the one learned) association and the actual output vector was computed when the first member of the association was presented.

162

more than once. If we then subtract the **g** out that arises from the synaptic interactions of the input **f** with the matrix, **A**, from the desired **g**, which is the correct association to be learned, we have a simple error correction procedure. Because both patterns are immediately present in the system in this procedure, this would be physiologically realizable.

Formally, instead of having the incremental change, $\Delta\mathbf{A}$, associating **f** and **g** proportional to $(\mathbf{gf}^T)$ the incremental change, $\Delta\mathbf{A}$, is now given by the proportionality

$$\Delta\mathbf{A} \propto (\mathbf{g} - \mathbf{g}_{out})\mathbf{f}^T$$

The actual output, $\mathbf{g}_{out}$, is given by

$$\mathbf{g}_{out} = \mathbf{Af}.$$

This learning rule is essentially the "Widrow–Hoff" rule, as described by Sutton and Barto (1981) in their recent review.

It is clear that the incremental matrix, $\Delta\mathbf{A}$, will be zero if the actual and desired outputs are identical, otherwise there will be a correction learned. Clearly, as $\mathbf{g}_{out}$ and **g** get close, learning will be less and less, suggesting convergence to equality. As can be easily shown, this rule is closely related to the best solution in the sense of linear regression.

A lot can be done with this rule analytically. (See Sutton & Barto, 1981, for references.) We did a simulation to check its behavior in practice, using the same kind of pairs of random vectors as in the previous section. As long as the number of random associations was less than the dimensionality, the convergence to "correct" association occurred. Table 8.1 gives values of the average cosine between **g** and $\mathbf{g}_{out}$ for different parameter. Even with only 20% of the matrix nonzero, after about 500 trials the average cosine was above .8 for 25 pairs of vectors. With 40% connectivity and 25 pairs there was essentially perfect fidelity of association. More nonzero matrix elements produced better behavior. This simulation, as is common with all our others on these systems was, robust. No parameter appeared critical, and failure was gradual in the sense that the average cosine gradually dropped as conditions became less favorable. Convergence to the final values was generally fairly rapid, with 10–30 presentations of each pair usually being enough to give asymptotic behavior.

The point of both these simulations is that these associative systems are not temperamental and they are quite resistant to variations in their parameters.

Feature Analysis and Categorization

What psychologists and, in particular, linguists mean by "feature" seems to be a kind of atom, out of which complex stimuli are made. Those interested in pattern recognition also speak about features like this.

TABLE 8.1
Test of Error Correction Procedure

# Associations	25		50		75		100	
% Connectivity	avg cos	pres	avg cos	pres	avg cos	pres	avg cos	pres
20	0.82	(5000)	0.42	(5000)	0.26	(5000)	0.20	(5000)
40	1.00	(300)	0.80	(5000)	0.53	(5000)	0.41	(5000)
60	1.00	(175)	1.00	(1875)	0.79	(5000)	0.61	(5000)
80	1.00	(125)	1.00	(775)	0.94	(5000)	0.80	(5000)
100	1.00	(90)	1.00	(420)	1.00	(1860)	0.94	(5000)

Note: Results of presentation of pairs of random vectors (normalized, with uniformly distributed elements of mean zero) to the associative system. The system learned according to the error correction rule described in the text. Pairs of vectors were presented at random. The percentage of connectivity refers to the percentage of nonzero elements in the synaptic connectivity matrix, values for which ranged from 20% to 100%. Dimensionality was 100.

The value "avg cos" gives the average cosine of angle between actual output of system and the associated output the system was trying to reproduce when the associated input is presented. The average is taken over all the pairs of random vectors to be associated. 1.00 is perfect fidelity of association.

The number in parentheses ("pres") gives the number of total presentations required to attain an average cosine of .99. A maximum of 5000 learning trials was used. If an average cosine of .99 or better was not attained, the value given is the value at 5000 presentations.

Suppose we have a perceptual task that requires the classification of an external stimulus into one or another of a set of categories. Recognizing a set of noises as a phoneme is one example, or a set of marks as a particular letter. Describing an event by a word, or recognizing that a particular tree is an oak is another, more complicated example, It should be appreciated that this is what a great deal of cognition is about and the ability to categorize appropriately is what gives language in particular and human cognition in general much of its power.

A very useful strategy for this task would be the following: Events of any complexity never recur exactly and may be embedded in a highly variable context. Suppose, however, that there were certain aspects of the particular item that were always present. If we looked for these aspects alone and ignored the other information as irrelevant, we could make efficient categorizations based on a much simplified set of information. These salient aspects of the stimulus set are called "features."

In linguistics, where the "distinctive feature" has a key role in phonetics, a feature might correspond to something like the presence or absence of vocal cord vibration, or of energy in certain frequency bands, or of a noiselike character to the stimulus, or a number of other acoustic aspects of the input.

These models are discussed in greater length in Anderson, et al. (1977) and Anderson and Mozer (1981).

Models for Feature Analysis

Our earlier discussion of neuronal selectivity is particularly relevant here. Features, as elementary aspects of the stimulus, seem particularly likely to correspond to the known single-unit selectivities found in the nervous system. One obvious example concerns recognition of written letters. Numerous feature sets have been published suggesting that letters are composed of oriented line segments like the cells known to exist in profusion in Area 17 of visual cortex.

There is a serious problem here. If one looks carefully at published data on selectivity of single cells, one rarely seems to find cells responding to stimuli with either the generality or the invariant properties expected of true "feature detectors." Typical Area 17 cells will respond to a number of aspects of the visual stimulus. Cells can be highly selective, but not as selective as required. It seems clear that features must correspond, to be useful, to somewhat more complex aspects of the stimulus. This is especially true in language, where proposed acoustic features are often complex in their acoustic description. We also note that there are very many more neurons than psychological or linguistic features; the discrepancy here is many orders of magnitude.

A Distributed Model for Features

Because we have been emphasizing the centrality of state vectors for models of nervous system organization, can we suggest a model based on state vectors for feature analysis? As we shall show, the answer is yes, and the resulting analysis sheds an interesting light on single-cell selectivity.

Let us consider what form a categorization model using state vectors would take. To avoid the necessity of a homunculus (an internal statistician) looking at the input data, to be consistent with our modeling approach, we must actually construct the categorization. For example, presentation of a number of different, complex, physical objects causes the vocal tract musculature, under the command of many motor neurons, to emit the word "table." This constant motor output pattern has been constructed in response to a variable input stimulus. Ideally, our neural system would not analyze the stimulus by breaking it into parts and computing on those parts in the traditional way, but could achieve the same end by simply emitting the appropriate output in the appropriate situation. We are far away from this ultimate goal, but the model that follows captures the beginnings of this project (Fig. 8.3).

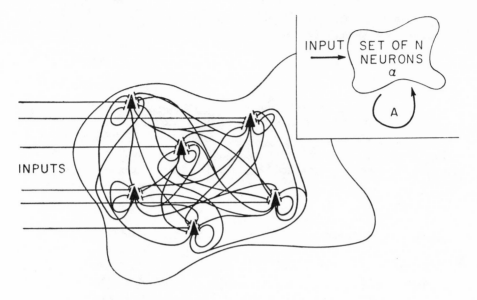

1. SET OF N NEURONS, α
2. EVERY NEURON IN α IS CONNECTED TO EVERY
   OTHER NEURON IN α THROUGH LEARNING
   MATRIX OF SYNAPTIC CONNECTIVITIES A

FIG. 8.3 A group of neurons feeds back on itself by way of modifiable synapses. Note the possibility of feedback of a cell onto itself. (From Anderson, Silverstein, Ritz, & Jones, 1977).

Let us at first consider a system very much like the simple associator we just discussed. Now, however, we will consider only a single set of neurons and let this set connect to itself by way of a set of lateral interconnections.

As a matter of anatomical fact, cortex contains an extensive set of connections of exactly this kind: the recurrent collateral system of cortical pyramids. This very extensive series of lateral connections means that one pyramid can influence others up to several millimeters away. It is not simple lateral inhibition because evidence suggests it is excitatory. (see Shepherd, 1979; Szentagothai, 1978).

Let us make the assumption that this set of lateral interconnections is capable of the kind of modification that gave rise to the interesting properties of the associative model. When a pattern of activity learns itself, the synaptic increment is given by

$$\Delta A(i, j) = \Delta A(j, i) \propto f(i)f(j).$$

The matrix **A** is closely related to the sample covariance matrix. This means that the kinds of results obtained in principal component analysis can hold and, as a result, the eigenvectors of the resulting matrix with the largest positive eigenvalues contain the largest amount of the variance of the system. If a set of items is to be discriminated, then these eigenvectors are the most useful for making discriminations among members of the set; this is what makes principal component analysis so useful.

This is a feedback system. The coefficient of feedback is set by the eigenvalue. Positive feedback will cause a relative enhancement of the eigenvectors with large positive eigenvalues. Because these are also the most useful parts of the stimulus for making discriminations among members of the set, we have a weighting that favors the most "useful" eigenvectors.

If we call these particular eigenvectors, the ones with large positive eigenvalues, "features," then we have a system that does what we want feature analysis to do.

We have here a demonstration of the powers and strategies of a parallel system. If this kind of weighting is desired, the resulting system, both theoretically and in computer simulation, is tremendously robust. However, it is not an analytical decomposition. At no point are the features themselves ever available, only a weighted sum. The system is fast, but perhaps not as flexible as a more analytical system. It is much more difficult to reprogram and debug.

Microfeatures and Macrofeatures

We now have a system where "features" are patterns of activity rather than selctive single cells. Yet clearly there must be a close relationship between the kinds of selectivities found in the single elementary units that make up the patterns of activities and the selectivities of the features. To avoid confusion, let us coin two ugly new words from a nice but ambigious old one: "feature."

Let us define a *microfeature* as the kind of selectivity shown by single cells. The microfeatures of visual cortex seem to be oriented line segments. There are very many of them in visual cortex and they change from cell to cell. When neuroscientists talk about features they are talking about microfeatures.

Let us define a *macrofeature* as the pattern of activity that corresponds to a particular perceptual feature. However this entity is a pattern of activity, a vector. Perception takes place by analysis in terms of macrofeatures. The vectors are made up of components that respond to microfeatures. When psychologists, linguists, and cognitive scientists talk about features they are talking about macrofeatures.

Feedback and Saturation

Let us make further modifications of the feedback system. We should carefully separate two aspects of the model we have just presented: the learning, and the dynamics. The feedback takes place in real time; macrofeature analysis is a dynamic process, provoked by a stimulus input.

Learning, change in strength of connection, takes place on a different time scale. Once the connections have been formed for a particular stimulus set, learning can cease, and the feedback system will continue to analyze the inputs in terms of the inputs. (This corresponds to the difference between programming, and running a program.)

We have investigated many variants of both processes. Let us describe a particularly simple approach. Suppose the response to the input pattern and the output of the feedback system interact significantly and have comparable time courses. We chose a very simple dynamics for our first modeling efforts. More complex dynamics ar now being studied.

Let $\mathbf{x}(t)$ denote the state vector at time t. Integer values are taken by t in the simulations because these were computer models. We assume there is no significant delay, therefore the activity at time $(t + 1)$ is assumed to be the sum of activity at time t and the activity of the feedback matrix on the activity at time t. Therefore we have the simple expression

$$\mathbf{x}(t + 1) = \mathbf{x}(t) + \mathbf{A}\mathbf{x}(t)$$
$$= (\mathbf{I} + \mathbf{A})\,\mathbf{x}(t)$$

where $\mathbf{I}$ is the identity matrix.

The Brain-State-in-a-Box

Unfortunately, all positive values of eigenvalue lead to activity growing without bound. We must discard the linearity of dynamics we have assumed. We need to keep the system from blowing up.

The simplest way of containing the activity is to observe that neurons have limits on their activities; they cannot fire faster than some frequency or slower than zero. Suppose we incorporate this in our model. A particular state vector is a point in a high-dimensional space. Putting limits on firing rate corresponds to putting allowable state vectors in a hypercube, leading to the nickname for this model of the "brain-state-in-a-box."

Our primary interest in the hypercube becomes the 2 to the Nth corners. Suppose we start off with an activity pattern receiving positive feedback. The vector lengthens until it reaches a wall of the box (i.e., a firing limit for one component). The vector will try to lengthen but cannot escape. It heads for a corner where it will remain if the corner is stable; not all corners are stable. If we allow decay, there are stable points outside corners, but many components of the state vector will still saturate. Figure 8.4 shows a sample two-dimensional system.

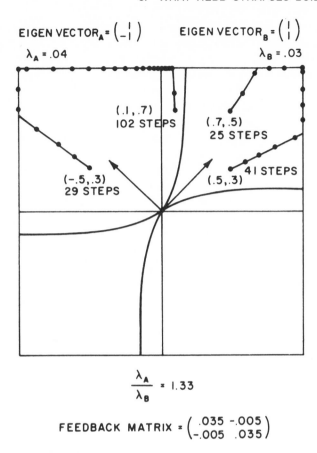

FIG. 8.4   Simple example of two-dimensional brain-state-in-a-box model. *x*- and *y*-axes correspond to activities in a two-neuron system. Feedback is applied through the feedback matrix, which has eigenvectors pointing toward corners and with eigenvalues as shown. Curved lines passing through the origin are the boundaries of equivalence regions corresponding to one or another corner. Dots are placed on trajectories every five iterations, and the total number of steps required to reach a corner is placed next to the starting point. (From Anderson & Silverstein, 1977).

Categorical Perception

The dynamics of this model gives rise to a categorical perceiver because it takes a set of initial points in a region of space and lumps them together in a single corner. We have produced a classification algorithm, where the state vector representing the categorization is the classification. We have constructed this categorization from the input, using distributed computation. There has been no analysis in the traditional sense.

Let us now do a performance test of the classifier, the third point on our list of requirements for organizational models of the nervous system. We have done a number of computer simulations of this algorithm. Let me briefly describe a large simulation I did last year with Mike Mozer. (Anderson & Mozer, 1981) Various aspects of this simulation have been replicated for other stimulus sets, with equivalent results.

For our large simulation we used capital letters. We coded uppercase letters into 117 element vectors. The coding was straightforward and was meant to be as much like the way the visual system codes stimuli as possible. Part of the vector was a point-for-point excitatory mapping of the visual stimulus with an accompanying inhibitory surround. The letters were placed on a 7 by 7 matrix and letters were drawn in what seemed to be a reasonable way. The surround could extend into a 9 by 9 grid, making 81 matrix elements. The other 36 elements were coded by looking for oriented line segments. The presence and orientation of line segments in these nine regions was coded by the response of orientation selective units, responding to the presence or absence of a line segment oriented at zero, 45, 90, and 135 degrees. Vectors were normalized, and the mean vector across the stimulus set was subtracted. This was done to avoid saturation of learning with the mean letter. The reason for this coding was to produce a first approximation to the multitude of ways the nervous system codes a sensory input.

In the learning phase of the simulation, letter vectors were presented at random. The feedback matrix was applied according to the previous equation for seven iterations. The final state, $\mathbf{x}$, was then learned according to the outer product learning rule (with η as the learning parameter),

$$\Delta \mathbf{A} = \eta \mathbf{x}^T$$

with one modification. We assumed that it was necessary to limit learning at some point. Our limitation assumption — there are many other possibilities — notes the final value of the cell's firing rate after seven iterations. If it is at a limit, then there is no change in the synaptic strengths of that cell, pre- or postsynaptically.

There is absolutely no instruction in this procedure. The system does not know if classification was fast or slow, correct or incorrect, or anything else. It seems obvious that even the most elementary feedback along these lines should improve results, as was demonstrated in a previous section for the simple associative model. Behavior of the system is very insensitive to the learning parameter. Simulations were made where the learning parameter varied over two orders of magnitude with no essential difference in behavior.

Results

The pattern of results we have now seen many times appeared here as well. At first, the system miscategorized different letters into particular corners, forming clumps of letters. With more trials the clumps separated, until at 5000 trials only "W" and "N," whose codings were extremely similar in this simulation, were classified together. At 10,000 learning trials, "W" and "N" were still classified together, but the simulation was halted.

One of the most interesting aspects of this system is that when we study the dynamics of classification, we find that speed of categorization increases as the system learns more. The system gets both faster and more accurate with experience.

Many of the most significant aspects of behavior of the system should appear in the structure of the eigenvectors and the eigenvalues. Because of their hypothesized closeness to the factors of factor analysis, we should be able to represent the letters as appropriately weighted sums of the first few eigenvectors and expect to find behavior very similar to that when all the eigenvectors are present. This is so.

If the letters are represented as the sum of the first 10 components, the resulting corners are very close to the complete set, though not exactly the same. Because the eigenvectors represent macrofeatures, one might wonder if there was any obvious "interpretation" of the eigenvectors with largest positive eigenvalue. Close scrutiny certainly did not reveal any obvious interpretations to us, at least not anything that looked like the nice lines and corners of published feature sets.

Connection with Single-Cell Selectivity

Suppose we consider the behavior and representation of single units in this simulation. Initially, the network is completely interconnected, every unit connected to every other unit. The stimulus set, by design, had positive or negative responses from virtually every element. Specificity is not built in. Also, the final state of the system is fully on or fully off, so there was no single-unit selectivity here either.

Does selectivity appear at the feature level? That is, what are the responses of the elements to features when they are first presented or when there is no feedback: responses to stimulus fragments? There are 117 model neurons. If we look at histograms of their relative representations in the eigenvectors we find considerable selectivity. Over all the 10 largest eigenvectors, about 100 of the 117 elements have little response to a given eigenvector. Some eigenvectors are represented by the vigorous response of only a few elements, whereas others have a larger amount of more uniformly responding cells. This pattern might be interpreted as showing considerable selectivity if turned up at the end of a microelectrode, but we should emphasize that in no case does this correspond to a single-element single-feature result, and the cumulative effect of the many small elements is quite substantial.

We can also look at the response of single elements. Do they respond to one and only one eigenvector or to several? Results here show a similar picture. Examples of extreme selectivity can be found, but most cells respond to more than one eigenvector.

It is clear that, with respect to the macrofeature vectors the system has developed, from an initially nonselective system, a moderate degree of selectivity. An enquiring neuroscientist might have interpreted such a pattern as evidence for grandmother cells, but the actual picture is much less clearcut.

Conclusion

We have discussed several things in this chapter. We tried to emphasize that to make models of brain organization we can and must proceed on several levels: structure, behavior, and performance.

We suggested that it was most useful to study patterns of activity shown simultaneously by many neurons. We suggested that developing models based on state vectors was the most likely way to make connections between system structure and system behavior.

We presented a simple model that took an elementary local learning asssumption and showed that it could serve as general purpose associator of state vectors. The model was functional with partial connectivity and could be "taught" to give very good accuracy of association when a correction procedure was used. We considered a variant of this model using lateral feedback. It was necessary to coin two new words "microfeature" and "macrofeature" to make clear the distinction between single unit selectivity studied by neurophysiologists and the technique of stimulus analysis held to exist by psychologists and linguists and called "feature analysis."

A large simulation of the feature model incorporating limits on neuron response (the "brain-state-in-a-box" model) showed the system could act as an acceptable, uninstructed categorizer. Model neurons developed moderate selectivities to macrofeature vectors.

These models also have important psychological implications, which are discussed at length elsewhere. (See Anderson, 1977; Anderson, 1983; Hinton & Anderson, 1981).

ACKNOWLEDGMENTS

The research presented here was supported with grants from the National Science Foundation (Grant BNS–79–23900) and the Alfred P. Sloan Foundation. The computing facilities of the Center for Cognitive Science, Brown University, received support from the National Science Foundation, The Alfred P. Sloan Foundation, and Digital Equipment Corporation.

REFERENCES

Anderson, J. A. Neural models with cognitive implications. In D. LaBerge & S. J. Samuels (Eds.), *Basic processes in reading: Perception and comprehension.* Hillsdale, N.J.: Lawrence Erlbaum Associates, 1977.

Anderson, J. A. Cognitive and psychological computation with neural models. *IEEE Transactions on Systems, Man, and Cybernetics,* 1983, *SMC-13,* 799-815.

Anderson, J. A., & Hinton, G. Models of information in the brain. In G. Hinton & J. A. Anderson (Eds.), *Parallel models of associative memory.* Hillsdale, N.J.: Lawrence Erlbaum Associates, 1981.

Anderson, J. A., & Mozer, M. Categorization and selective neurons. In G. Hinton & J. A. Anderson (Eds.), *Parallel models of associative memory.* Hillsdale, N.J.: Lawrence Erlbaum Associates, 1981.

Anderson, J. A., & Silverstein, J. W. Reply to Grossberg. *Psychological Review,* 1978, *85,* 597-603.

Anderson, J. A., Silverstein, J. W., Ritz, S. A., & Jones, R. S. Distinctive features, categorical perception, and probability learning: Some applications of a neural model. *Psychological Review,* 1977, *84,* 413-451.

Hebb, D. O. *The organization of behavior.* New York: Wiley, 1949.

Hinton, G., & Anderson, J. A. (Eds.) *Parallel models for associative memory.* Hillsdale, N.J.: Lawrence Erlbaum Associates, 1981.

Kohonen, T. *Associative memory: A system theoretic approach.* Berlin: Springer-Verlag, 1977.

Shepherd, G. M. *The synaptic organization of the brain.* (2nd ed.). New York: Oxford, 1979.

Sutton, R. S., & Barto, A. G. Toward a modern theory of adaptive networks: Expectation and prediction. *Psychological Review,* 1981, *88,* 135-170.

Szentagothai, J. Specificity versus (quasi) randomness in cortical connectivity. In M. A. B. Brazier & H. Petsche (Eds.), *Architectonics of the cerebral cortex.* New York: Raven Press, 1978.

9 Neuron Selectivity: Single Neuron and Neuron Networks

L. N. Cooper
P. Munro
C. Scofield
Physics Dept. of Brown University and
Center for Neural Science

In the formulation of theories describing neural processing of any kind, certain elements common to all such theories must be considered, for example the connectivity of the neuronal network. Consider a network (Fig. 9.1) in which one population of neurons d projects to another population c. The net connectivity between the jth cell of the input population (d_j) and the ith output cell (c_i) is given by the value M_{ij}. A typical connectivity, M_{ij}, represents the net influence of several synapses, both in parallel and in series, both excitatory and inhibitory, possibly involving interneurons. M_{ij} represents the efficacy of an "ideal synapse" (Nass & Cooper, 1975), a useful concept to the mathematician, but one that falls short of ideal in the anatomist's eyes. The idea is that each input axon firing frequency is converted to some net postsynaptic membrane depolarization in a given cell in the target population (c) and eventually will influence the firing of the cell. Mathematically speaking, the synaptic array M *operates* on the stimulus vector d, producing the response vector c (Equation 1).

$$c = Md \tag{1}$$

These same assumptions have been described in two other chapters (Anderson; Kohonen). In effect they have said that the connectivity matrix M can evolve to function as a memory. By "memory" we generally mean that the synaptic strengths M_{ij} contain information in that they affect "appropriate responses" in the postsynaptic population c to certain patterns of afferent activity. Rigorous mathematical theorems can be proven to show that such memory systems work. Kohonen (1977) used facial photographs encoded

175

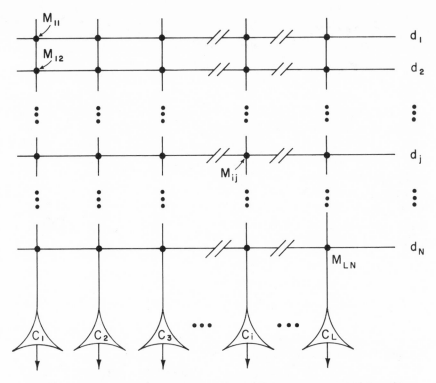

FIG. 9.1   Schematic representation of an $L \times N$ array of ideal synaptic junctions. The value M_{ij} gives the net influence of the jth afferent on the ith cell.

into a string of darkness (brightness) values, each representing a small element of the visual field. The coded information from *each pattern* is distributed over *all synaptic junctions* in the network. This example is a beautifully graphic demonstration of what is meant by a *distributed memory*. This idea has the important quality that if any small portion of these junctions is lost, no specific faces are lost — rather the signal-to-noise ratio is reduced.

The principles that determine the evolution of a synaptic network with experience have to be formulated carefully to yield a system that is capable of both extracting information from the environment and accessing that same information at a later time. Ideally, the postsynaptic population c will learn to respond appropriately to inputs d depending on whether or not similar patterns have already been presented and, if so, in what context. Various types of modification rules yield memories that are suited to a variety of tasks. Over the last several years our group has developed a model of binocular orientation-selective cells in visual cortex by refining a set of equations for synaptic plasticity (Bienenstock, Cooper, & Munro, 1982; Cooper, Liberman, & Oja, 1979; Nass & Cooper, 1975) and is based on a diverse collection of physiological data.

EXPERIMENTAL DATA

Since the original work by Hubel and Wiesel (1959) that led to the realization that visual cortical cells respond in a highly specific fashion to visual stimuli, researchers have extended their studies to the development of this specificity in the newborn animal. Michel Imbert and his collaborators (Imbert & Buisseret, 1975) have classified visually responsive cells into three groups — aspecific, immature, and specific — according to their response properties and receptive field arrangements (Fig. 9.2). Aspecific cells are characterized by rather indiscriminant responses to circular stimuli moving in any direction across their receptive fields. The receptive field is usually rather large in size and circular in shape. Immature cells are more highly tuned in their response; they characteristically respond best to a correctly oriented rectilinear stimulus moving across the receptive field, and there is always an orientation for the stimulus that will evoke a negligible response. Their receptive fields are large, but more rectangular than the receptive fields of the aspecific cells. The most discriminant of all cells, the specific cells, show a sharp response to an optimal orientation of the stimulus and are much less responsive to other orientations. These cells have receptive fields that are

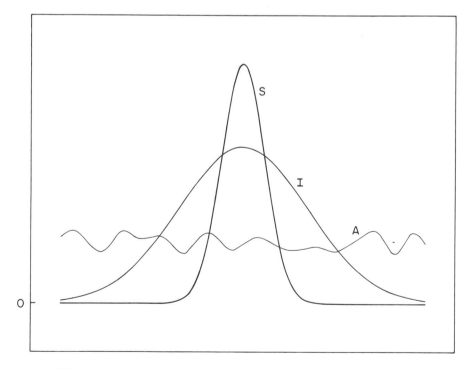

FIG. 9.2   Examples of aspecific (A), immature (I), and specific (S) response curves.

smaller in size than those of the two previous cell classes and are rectangular in shape.

The evolution of these different cell types has been studied for kittens raised in different visual environments (Fregnac, 1978; Fregnac & Imbert, 1977, 1978). The results for kittens raised in a normal visual environment (NR) and for those raised in complete darkness (DR) from the first or second day of age are compared in Figs. 9.3 and 9.4. This data indicates that in the earliest stages of development there are some cells present that exhibit specific cell properties. However, visual experience is critical in the development of these cells. The normally reared animals show a pronounced increase in the number of specific cells relative to aspecific cells, whereas dark-reared animals show just the opposite. The high degree of malleability of cortical cells in this critical period from about Day 17 to Day 70 is illustrated in Fig. 9.5. We see that as little as 6 hours of visual experience at 42 days of age can dramatically alter the ratio of specific to aspecific and immature cells (Buisseret, Gary-Bobo, & Imbert, 1978).

In addition, ocular dominance appears to depend on visual experience. It is found that before the age of 21 days, independent of visual experience, most immature and specific cells are driven optimally by the eye contralateral to the hemisphere in which they are located. After 3 weeks of age, normally reared animals exhibit a significant increase in binocularly driven cells (Fregnac & Imbert, 1978). This result is also found for animals that are dark reared (Blakemore & Mitchell, 1973; Blakemore & Van Sluyters, 1975; Buisseret & Imbert, 1976; Fregnac & Imbert, 1978; Imbert & Buisseret, 1975;

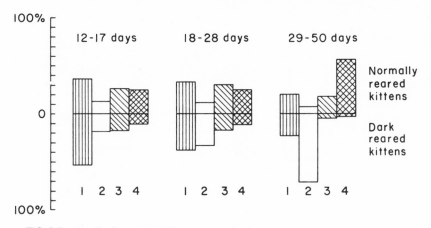

FIG. 9.3   Distribution of the different types of cells in three age groups in the normally reared kittens (upper part) and in the dark-reared kittens (lower part). The ordinate is normalized so that the heights are the percentages of cells in the various function groups. Type 1, nonactivatable (□); 2, nonspecific (▥); 3, immature (▨); 4, specific (▨). (From Fregnac & Imbert, 1977, 1978.)

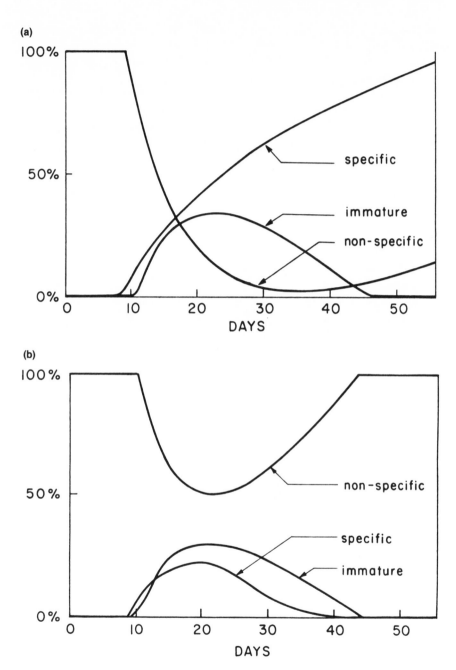

FIG. 9.4 Evolution of the development of the various specificity groups in cats raised (a) normally and (b) in total darkness. The results are based on an unweighted regression analysis of 1050 cells (From Fregnac, 1978.)

Leventhal & Hirsch, 1980). However, in animals whose eyelids have been sutured at birth (and thus deprived of binocular pattern vision, BD), a higher proportion of selective cells are found compared to dark-reared animals and the proportion of binocular cells is less than normal (Blakemore & Van Sluyters, 1975; Kratz & Spear, 1976; Leventhal & Hirsch, 1977; Watkins, Wilson, & Sherman, 1978; Wiesel & Hubel, 1965).

Finally, one of the clearest examples of the dependence of cortical development on the environment occurs when an animal is raised with one eye in competitive advantage over the other. When monocular lid suture (MD) is

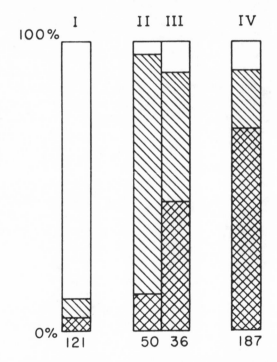

FIG. 9.5   Distribution, in percentage, of the three types of visual cortical units (Area 17) recorded after 6 hours of visual exposure for 6-week-old dark-reared kittens. Columns: I, dark-reared kittens; IV, normally reared kittens. During 6 hours of exposure, conditions were: in II and III, freely moving; in III, 12 hours in the dark followed the 6 hours of exposure. Numbers of visual cells recorded are given under each column. Specific cells (▨) are activated by oriented stimuli within a sharp angle (< 60°). Immature cells (▧) are activated by oriented stimuli within a larger angle (< 150°). Nonspecific cells (□) are activated by nonoriented stimuli moving in any direction. A statistical analysis reveals no significant difference in the percentages of immature and specific units in between columns III and IV. Therefore it may be that for a 6-week-old dark-reared kitten, a 6-hour exposure to visual input followed by 12 hours in the dark is sufficient to produce a distribution of cortical cells similar to that of normally reared animals. (From Buisseret, Gary-Bobo, & Imberg, 1978.)

performed during the critical period, a rapid loss of binocularity to the profit of the open eye occurs (Wiesel & Hubel, 1963, 1965). If the sutures are reversed (RS), the closed eye opened and the experienced eye closed, it is possible to observe a complete reversal of ocular dominance (Blakemore & Van Sluyters, 1974).

FORMULATION OF THE THEORY

Of the characteristic properties described in the preceding section for stages of neuronal development in visual cortex, this theory deals primarily with the development of selectivity. The pattern environment available to the neuron consists of impulses directly associated with a specific receptive field on the retina and secondary lateral influences from cortical cells having different primary receptive fields that may overlap to varying degrees. One can easily imagine how synaptic delays can account for the translation of a spatiotemporal pattern such as a moving bar to a near simultaneous, purely spatial pattern of postsynaptic potentials at a neuron's dendritic surface. Hence, the notion of a visual stimulus should be considered in its most general sense.

Refraining from choosing *completely ad hoc* assumptions, we first consider what aspects of a given synapse's environment might influence its development. Changes in the physical structure of either the presynaptic or postsynaptic elements or the cleft itself, as well as the chemistry of the synapse's immediate neighborhood come to mind as primary candidates. Of course consideration of proposed biochemical mechanisms (Changeaux et al., 1973) can be most useful at this stage of model development.

Let us begin developing our model with a formal statement of the functional dependence of dm/dt (Equation 2). Namely, we assume here that the change in efficacy of a give synapse depends on the efficacy itself, both the presynaptic and postsynaptic activities, as well as a time average of the postsynaptic activity. Global factors may well play a strong modulatory role (see for example Kasamatsu & Pettigrew, 1976, 1979), but we do not consider them here

$$\dot{m} = \dot{m}(m, d, c, \bar{c}) \tag{2}$$

Two linear assumptions are made in this model. First, the transfer function (Equation 3a), or input–output relation, is simply an inner product. More complicated functions have been tested and do not seem to have a qualitative influence on the results as long as they are monotonically increasing in both m and d. The modification function (Equation 3b) includes the second linear assumption, namely that dm/dt is linear in d. Neglecting the second term, we see that the model relies on the premise that the change in the synaptic vector is parallel to the input, hence the response characteristics of the cell are influenced for that input more than any other possible stimulus of the same magnitude.

$$c = \sum_i m_i d_i \tag{3a}$$

$$\dot{m}_i = \phi(c, \bar{c})d_i \tag{3b}$$

This model is predicated on the notion that if $\phi > 0$ for a given input and the evoked response, then the m_{ij} change such that the cell's response to a future presentation of the same stimulus is enhanced. This idea was first put forward by Hebb (1949), so we will term such modification *Hebbian*. Similarly a stimulus–response combination yielding a negative value for phi decreases the cell's affinity to that stimulus (*anti-Hebbian*). The conditions on ϕ are illustrated by the arbitrary function in Fig. 9.6.

Because we are modeling cells that become highly selective, we design a system that weakens responses to weak patterns and strengthens responses to strong ones. The strength of a neuron's response to a pattern is evaluated relative to a time-varying threshold value (θ) intrinsic to the cell, at which ϕ vanishes. This "floating" threshold is linked to the expectation value of the cell's response evaluated with respect to the stimulus environment. If the time scale for synaptic modification is sufficiently larger than the usual duration of an input presentation, then this expectation value is close to a time average.

If the threshold could not vary in time, the system would require some very specific assumptions (Cooper et al., 1979) in order to account for the highly tuned cells observed in visual cortex. By allowing theta to vary with the aver-

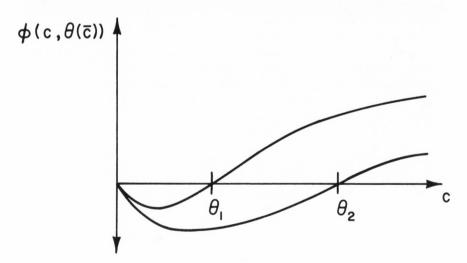

FIG. 9.6   The modulatory function $\phi[c, \theta(\bar{c})]$ is shown for two values of $\theta(\bar{c})$. As $\bar{c}$ increases, so does θ. The modification is (anti-) Hebbian ((anti-) parallel to the input vector d if the evoked response c is greater (less) than θ.

age response in a faster-than-linear fashion, the response characteristics evolve to maximum selectivity over the input environment. This spatiotemporal modification scheme forces theta and the nontrivial response values toward a common value such that the threshold is driven between them. When this occurs the response values below theta decrease toward zero and theta "overtakes" the other values, which have begun to increase. Eventually only a small subset of the stimuli drives the cell above the modification threshold. In certain cases (see Appendix), it has been proved that maximum selectivity is attained. Barring situations where some inputs have negative inner products (Bienenstock, 1980), computer simulations indicate that the neuron is always driven to a maximally selective state.

The simple case of a neuron driven by two equiprobable two-dimensional stimuli provides a good example for examining these properties of the model. The input environment consists of two linearly independent vectors, d^1 and d^2, which are normalized and have a nonnegative inner product. They can be represented in a common vector space with the synaptic state vector m, because each afferent (a component in each d^i) corresponds to a unique ideal synapse (a component in m). We begin by seeking points that are candidates for stationary final states (fixed points); we then look at the behavior of the system relative to these points. If we assume that the synaptic weights change slowly relative to the frequency of stimulus presentation, then we can assume that a fixed point represents any state for which the net modification induced by the two patterns is zero. Because the patterns are independent, dm/dt must be zero for *each* stimulus.

Let $\theta = \bar{c}^2$ give the threshold value for the phi function. We seen then that the locus of points for which $\phi = 0$ for a given input (Fig. 9.7) is the union of two loci, namely a line corresponding to $c = 0$ (Equation 4a) and a parabola corresponding to $c = \theta$ (Equation 4b). The intersections of these isoclines give the four fixed points, at which both patterns must give $\phi = 0$. We define the order of a fixed point, s, to be the number (0, 1, or 2, in this example) of patterns that yield the response $c = \theta$. Figure 9.7 divides the space into four regions, characterized by the sign of phi attributed to each pattern. Thus we see that the asymptotically stable final states are *fixed points of maximum selectivity*. An example of local stability analysis is given in the Appendix.

$$m \cdot d^i = 0 \qquad i = 1, 2 \tag{4a}$$

$$m \cdot d^i = (m \cdot \bar{d})^2 \qquad i = 1, 2 \tag{4b}$$

SIMULATIONS OF BINOCULAR INTERACTION

The simulated behavior of neurons in visual cortex with binocular connectivity is illustrated in Fig. 9.8. The seemingly inconsistent experimental results (MD versus BD) are faithfully reproduced by computer simulation ac-

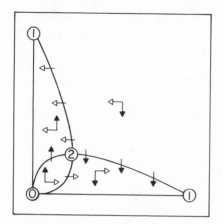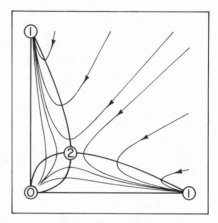

FIG. 9.7   The state space of a two-synapse cell in a two-pattern environment is shown. (a). The directions of change in the state m as a result of each input are shown. Each fixed point is labeled by its order s. One can see that along the isoclines, $\phi = 0$ with respect to one of the patterns. The $s = 2$ point is a saddle point: It attracts trajectories from some directions, but repels them in others, so it is not stable. The $s = 0$ point repels all nearby states. Hence only the $s = 1$ points are stable. (b). Some sample trajectories are shown with the isoclines (bold).

cording to the model outlined here. Thus this theory gives one explanation that resolves the paradox. Each of these paradigms was tested in both deterministic and stochastic simulation algorithms over several pattern sets. The model withstood considerable noisy input, indeed successful simulation of some paradigms (RS in particular) *required* that a noiselike component accompany the "pure" inputs.

Binocular interactions do not play a special role in understanding the behavior of this theory with respect to either binocular deprivation or (correlated) normal rearing. That is, due to idealizing assumptions (for example, disparity between left and right inputs is *not* considered), these two cases drive the model neuron just as it would be driven if its connections were strictly monocular. Binocular stimuli presented in NR simulations were exactly correlated so that each pattern incident to the left-eye synapses was consistently accompanied by a corresponding pattern to the right-eye synapses. So each binocular input enjoys a one-to-one correspondence with a particular input to either eye. The left and right components of each pair used here are identical, hence the cell tunes to the same pattern in each eye (Fig. 9.8a). Binocularly deprived input environments consisted of stimulus components uniformly distributed over some range with zero mean. In this case (BD), the average response of the cell is null and so phi is always nonnegative, resulting in the synaptic state modifying randomly (Fig. 9.8b).

The development of a neuron receiving patterned input from only one eye (and uniform noise from the other) is interesting. The naive prediction integrating the results in the foregoing paragraph is incorrect. Namely, even

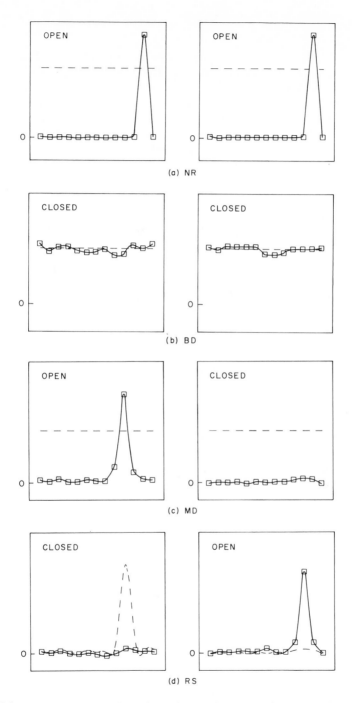

FIG. 9.8   Results of machine simulation of neuron development in four experimental paradigms: (a) Normal Rearing; (b) Binocular Deprivation; (c) Monocular Deprivation; and (d) Reverse Suture. Each figure shows the response versus orientation of the test stimuli to each eye both before (dashed) and after (solid) a period of plastic development.

though the response curve seeks maximum selectivity with respect to the open eye, the response to the other eye does *not* fluctuate randomly. Rather, as in the laboratory, the neuron becomes nonresponsive to inputs to the deprived eye (Fig. 9.8c). Asymptotic convergence to this state is assured *regardless of the initial state*. Thus the theoretical implications for the RS paradigm are straightforward: A monocularly deprived neuron, having reached a monocular selective state, is driven to another monocular selective state preferring the *newly opened eye* upon reversal of suture (Fig. 9.8d).

The monocular results rely on some activity, albeit purely random, to be present in the afferents from the closed eye. Such noise may be due to diffuse light through the eyelid or spontaneous firing of LGN and/or retinal neurons. As a neuron becomes selective with respect to the open eye, those few patterns that are preferred give a response near threshold whereas the other patterns give a much lower response. In either case phi is near zero. Noise accompanying a preferred pattern drives the neuron beyond the modification threshold, so the deprived synapses grow stronger. However, the opposite effect weakens the synapses when "uninteresting" patterns are presented. A mathematical demonstration of this argument is given in the Appendix.

NEW DIRECTIONS

So far we have been discussing selectivity on the single-unit level. However, cortical anatomy suggests that the geniculocortical component of the afferents to a cell is a small fraction of those afferents (Hornung & Garey, 1981). Thus it is very likely that cortico–cortical inputs play an important role in the development of neuron selectivity (Creutzfeldt, Kuhnt, & Benevento, 1974; Sillito, 1975). The development of selectivity then might be viewed as a many-neuron problem.

Formulation of the many-neuron problem raises several issues. These may be classified into three broad categories. The first concerns relevant cortical anatomy. Neuroanatomical studies have provided extensive detail. We would like to include details relevant to the development of selectivity, yet keep the model to a manageable complexity. Second, the problem of response dynamics needs to be examined. The presence of cortico–cortical loops could lead to "resonance" effects in the response of a cell to a pattern. Thus the transfer function of the cell population must be more carefully defined than the single-cell case (see Equation 3a). Two possible solutions are: (1) cortical activity rapidly settles before the afferent message changes; and (2) cortical response to a pattern decays rapidly (Bienenstock et al., 1982). The final class of problems concerns the evolution of synaptic strengths. Physiological studies have yet to clarify which cell types develop stimulus selectivity. Thus we need to make assumptions about the evolution of geniculocortical synapses on inhibitory and excitatory cells. In addition, the role of plasticity in intracortical synapses is not clear.

The many-neuron problem has been treated before by other researchers. Von der Malsburg (1973) chose an anatomy of two cell types corresponding to excitatory and inhibitory cells. In his model, the two cell types were distributed equally but only the excitatory cells had geniculocortical afferents. The problem of response dynamics was solved according to alternative (1) in the preceding paragraph. Finally, von der Malsburg chose an intracortical circuitry in which a cell received static synapses that were short-range excitatory and long-range inhibitory.

Since this work, further experimental studies have emphasized the role of cortical inhibition in neuron selectivity (Sillito, 1975). However, evidence suggests that both inhibitory and excitatory cells receive geniculate afferents (Davis & Sterling, 1979). Our model uses a circuitry incorporating excitatory and inhibitory cells that both receive geniculate input. We assume alternative (2) already mentioned: Only monosynaptically and disynaptically mediated components of the geniculate message are integrated to give a cell's response. One of the results of incorporating a "first-order anatomy" into the many-neuron problem has been a resolution of the "ideal synapse" into separate excitatory and inhibitory synapses. It can be shown that under proper conditions on the intracortical inhibitory synapses, and assuming a nonselective inhibitory cell, excitatory cells that evolve according to Equation 3b will reach a state maximally selective with respect to their own individual environments. Thus, with respect to corticocortical connectivity, selectivity appears to depend more on inhibition than it does on excitation. Further work on the precise spatial relationships and evolution equations of the intracortical circuitry is necessary before the mechanisms specifying global cortical properties will be fully understood.

APPENDIX

The function $\phi(c, \bar{c})$ that describes the postsynaptic effect on the evolution of the synaptic efficacies has zeros at $c = 0$ and at $c = \bar{c}^p$. For those values of c, the synaptic strengths will not change. The values of m for which $\phi = 0$ when $d \neq 0$, are called fixed points. The fixed points of m-space can be classified according to the following criteria: A fixed point of index s is a point in m-space for which $m^*_i d^j = (m^*_i d)^p = \mu^{(s)}$, with $d^i \epsilon \, \mathscr{D}^\mu = \{ d^1, ..., d^s\}$ and $m^* \cdot d^i = 0$ for $d^i \epsilon \, \mathscr{D}^\circ = \{d^{s+1}, ..., d^k\}$.

The stability of a fixed point will be investigated, rather informally, by examining the time dependance of m if it is perturbed from the fixed point, m^*. A point is unstable if after a small perturbation $m = m^* + x$, ($|x| << |m^*|$), m evolves away from m^*. A point is stable if m returns to m^* after the perturbation.

Under proper restrictions on ϕ, we can assume that ϕ is a linear function of its argument for m near a fixed point. Thus for c near zero, $\phi(c, \bar{c}) \sim -\alpha_{\bullet}, c$, and for c near $\bar{c}^p$, $\phi(c, \bar{c}) \sim \alpha_{\mu}(c - \bar{c}^p)$. In the special case of $\bar{c}$ equal to zero, we assume that $\phi(c, 0) \sim \alpha c^2$. Where we define $\alpha_0 = \left.\dfrac{-\delta\phi}{\delta c}\right|_{c=0}$, $\alpha_{\mu} = \left.\dfrac{\delta\phi}{\delta c}\right|_{c=\bar{c}^p}$, and $\alpha = \left.\dfrac{\delta^2\phi}{\delta c^2}\right|_{\substack{c=0 \\ \bar{c}=0}}$. These assumptions greatly simplify the analysis of the local stability of a fixed point.

The environment of the cell is assumed to consist of K linearly independent vectors $\mathscr{D} \equiv \{d^1, ..., d^k\}$. Thus we define the average vector:

$$\bar{d} = 1/k \sum_{l=1}^{k} d^l.$$

Then for $d^i \epsilon \mathscr{D}^o$, $d^i \epsilon \mathscr{D}^{\mu}$:

$$m^* \cdot d^i = 0$$
$$m^* \cdot d^j = (m^* \cdot \bar{d})^2 = \mu^{(s)}.$$

With $\mu^{(s)} = (K/s)^2$ for $s > 0$.
and $\mu^{(0)} = 0$ for $s = 0$. Here we have specialized to $p = 2$.

The change in the synaptic strengths as a result of these vectors entering is:

$$\dot{m} = -\alpha_0(m \cdot d^i)d^i, \qquad d^i \epsilon \mathscr{D}^o$$
$$\dot{m} = +\alpha_{\mu}(m \cdot d^j - (m \cdot \bar{d})^2)d^j, \qquad d^j \epsilon \mathscr{D}^{\mu}.$$

m is very near the fixed point, so that $m = m^* + x$. If $\mathscr{D}$ forms a complete set (i.e., $K = N$) then we can expand x in the set $\mathscr{D}$:

$$x = \sum_{l=1}^{k} x_l d^l.$$

Thus the evolution of the perturbation is given by ($\dot{m} = \dot{x}$):

$$\dot{x} = -\alpha_0(x \cdot d^i)d^i$$
$$\dot{x} = -\alpha_{\mu}(x \cdot d)d^j + O(x^2)$$

where $d = d^j(2/s - 1) + 2/s \sum_{l \neq j}^{k} d^l$ for $s > 0$.

If $s = 0$ then all the d's belong to $\mathscr{D}^o$ and

$$\dot{x} = \alpha(x \cdot d^i)^2 d^i, \qquad \text{for } i = 1, 2, ..., K.$$

Now $x = \sum_{l=1}^{k} x_l d^l$. Thus $\dot{x} = \sum_{l=1}^{k} \dot{x}_l d^l$. For the K linearly independent vectors, the coefficient of each vector must vanish separately.

$$\dot{x}_i = -\alpha_0(x \cdot d^i)$$
$$\dot{x}_j = -\alpha_{\mu}(x \cdot d),$$

for $s = 0$: $\dot{x}_i = \alpha(x \cdot d^i)^2$.

Now we specialize to the simplest environment. Consider $\mathscr{D} = \{d^1, ..., d^k\}$ a set of $K = N$ linearly independent and orthonormal vectors. Then:

$$\dot{x}_i = -\alpha_0 x_i$$
$$\dot{x}_j = -\alpha_\mu(2/s - 1)x_j - \alpha_\mu 2/s \sum_q' x_q,$$

and for $s = 0$: $\dot{x}_i = \alpha(x_i)^2$.

where $\sum_q'$ means a sum over all q such that $d^q \in \mathscr{D}^\mu$.

Thus we see immediately that for $s = 0$, the perturbation x grows faster than exponentially, and m^* is an unstable fixed point. If $s > 0$, then $x_i = x_i(o)e^{-\alpha_0 t}$ and those components of the perturbation along the vectors for which $m^* \cdot d = 0$ will decay exponentially. What of the components of x along the "preferred" vectors for which $m^* \cdot d = (m^* \cdot \bar{d})^2$? Solving the second equation gives for $s = 1$ and $\alpha_\bullet \neq \alpha_\mu$:

$$x_j(t) = [x_j(0) - \frac{2 \alpha_\mu}{\alpha_0 - \alpha_\mu} X]e^{-\alpha_\mu t} + \frac{2 \alpha_\mu}{\alpha_0 - \alpha_\mu} Xe^{-\alpha_0 t}.$$

And for the special case of $\alpha_0 = \alpha_\mu$:

$$x_j(t) = [x_j(0) - 2\alpha_0 Xt]e^{-\alpha_0 t}.$$

We have made the definition that $X = \sum_q' x_q(0)$. Thus for $s = 1$, all components of the perturbation will vanish as t tends to ∞. The $s = 1$ point, that point for which $c = \bar{c}^2$ for one pattern and $c = 0$ for all other patterns, is a stable point.

Consider now $s = 2$. For this value of s, two patterns give a nonzero response, and all others give a zero response. Then $\mathscr{D}^\mu = \{d^1, d^2\}$ and $\mathscr{D}^\circ = \{d^3, ..., d^k\}$. The solutions of the differential equations for the components of x along d^1 and d^2 are (for $\alpha_\bullet \neq \alpha_\mu$):

$$x_1(t) = \frac{1}{2}[x_1(0) - x_2(0)]e^{\alpha_0 t} + \frac{1}{2}[x_1(0) + x_2(0)$$
$$- \frac{2 \alpha_\mu}{\alpha_0 - \alpha_\mu} X]e^{-\alpha_\mu t} + \frac{\alpha_\mu}{\alpha_0 - \alpha_\mu} e^{-\alpha_0 t},$$

$$x_2(t) = \frac{1}{2}[x_2(0) - x_1(0)]e^{\alpha_0 t} + \frac{1}{2}[x_2(0) + x_1(0)$$
$$- \frac{2 \alpha_\mu}{\alpha_0 - \alpha_\mu} X]e^{-\alpha_\mu t} + \frac{\alpha_\mu}{\alpha_0 - \alpha_\mu} e^{-\alpha_0 t},$$

and for $\alpha_0 = \alpha_\mu$:

$$x_1(t) = \frac{1}{2}[x_1(0) - x_2(0)]e^{\alpha_0 t} + \frac{1}{2}[x_1(0) + x_2(0) - \alpha_0 Xt]e^{-\alpha_0 t},$$

$$x_2(t) = [x_2(0) - x_1(0)]e^{\alpha_0 t} + [x_2(0) + x_1(0) - \alpha_0 Xt]e^{-\alpha_0 t},$$

Thus only in the special case of $x_1(0) = x_2(0)$ will the $s = 2$ point be stable. However this means that if the perturbation is only sightly off the line in m-space on which $x_1 = x_2$, then the perturbation will grow rapidly. This simply means that the $s = 2$ point is a saddle point. Further analysis for $s \geq 2$ yields similar results; for $s \geq 2$, the fixed points are unstable. Our linear analysis indicates that for the case of an orthonormal environment, only the $s = 1$ point is stable asymptotically.

These same methods may be used to illustrate the correlation between ocular dominance and selectivity in the monocular deprived environment. Following the arguments presented in Bienenstock et al. (1982), we consider an MD environment specified by the circular environment d_r for the right eye and n a "pure noise vector" for the left eye. We now assume the cell has evolved to the state given by $\phi(m_r^*, 0)$ where m_r^* is a stable selective state in the environment d_r. As before, we consider a perturbation from the fixed point; the state of the cell now is given by $\phi(m_r^* + x_r, x_l)$. The perturbation then evolves according to (where the noise is assumed to have zero mean):

$$\dot{x}_r = \phi(m_r^* \cdot d_r + x_r \cdot d_r + x_l \cdot n, \; m^* \cdot \vec{d}_r + x_r \cdot \vec{d}_r)d_r$$
$$\dot{x}_l = \phi(m_r^* \cdot d_r + x_r \cdot d_r + x_l \cdot n, \; m_r^* \cdot \vec{d}_r + x_r \cdot \vec{d}_r)n.$$

The stability of the equation for x_r has already been assumed in the conditions on m_r^*. The equation for x_l is analyzed by dividing the right eye inputs into those for which $\phi(m_r \cdot d_r, m_r \cdot d_r)$ is far from zero (either above or below) and those for which $\phi(m_r \cdot d_r, m_r \cdot d_r) = 0$. For those vectors in the first class, the sign of ϕ is determined by d_r alone, hence the equation for x_l is the equation of a random walk. Those vectors in the second class elicit a response near the threshold θ, or near zero. Using the methods already described, it is easy to see that vectors with a response near θ cause the perturbation to evolve according to:

$$\dot{x}_l \sim \alpha_\mu (x_l \cdot n)n$$

and those for which $m_r^* \cdot d_r \cong 0$ cause the perturbation to evolve like:

$$\dot{x}_l \sim -\alpha_0 (x_l \cdot n)n$$

where α_o and α_μ are defined above. Finally, averaging these equations (the distribution of n is assumed symmetric with respect to x_l) yields, respectively

$$\dot{x}_l \sim \alpha_\mu \overline{n_0^2} \, x_l$$
$$\dot{x}_l \sim -\alpha_o \overline{n_0^2} \, x_l$$

where $\overline{n_0^2}$ is the average squared magnitude of the noise input to a single synapse from the closed eye.

Now for the case of K linearly independent vectors defining the environment d_r, only vectors of the second class enter the system after $(m_r^*, 0)$ has been reached. Also, for m_r^* a stable selective state (i.e., $s = 1$), only one vector of d_r will elicit a response near threshold. Thus the results above show that only one input will cause the perturbation to grow and all others tend to return the state of the cell to (m_r^*, 0). For the general environment, the more selective m_r^* is with respect to d_r, the greater the number of inputs that will drive ($m_r^* + x_r$, x_l) to (m_r^*, 0). This linear analysis then allows us to conclude that under proper conditions on ϕ and (d_r, n), (Bienenstock et al., 1982), the state (m_r^*, 0) is stable on the average and the fluctuation of x_l due to 'preferred' patterns is smaller for more selective m_r^*.

ACKNOWLEDGEMENTS

This work was supported by the U.S. Office of Naval Research under contract N00014-81-K-0136 and by the A. P. Sloan Foundation.

REFERENCES

Bienenstock, E. L. "A Theory of Development of Neuronal Selectivity", Ph.D. Thesis, Division of Applied Mathmatics and Center for Neural Science, L. N. Cooper, Thesis Supervisor, June 1980.

Bienenstock, E. L., Cooper, L. N., & Munro, P. W. Theory for the development of neuron selectivity: Orientation selectivity and binocular interaction in visual cortex. *Jour. of Neurosci.*, 1982, *2*, 32–48.

Blakemore, C., & Mitchell, D. E. Environmental modification of the visual cortex and the neural basis of learning and memory. *Nature*, 1973, *241*, 467.

Blakemore, C., & Van Sluyters, R. C. Reversal of the physiological effects of monocular deprivation in kittens: Further evidence for a sensitive period. *J. Physiol.* (London), 1974, *237*, 195–216.

Blakemore, C., & Van Sluyters, R. C. Innate and environmental factors in the development of the kitten's visual cortex. *J. Physiol.* (London), 1975, *248*, 663–716.

Buisseret, P., Gary-Bobo, E., & Imbert, M. Ocular motility and recovery of orientational properties of visual cortex neurons in dark reared kittens. *Nature*, 1978, *272*, 816–817.

Buisseret, P., & Imbert, M. Visual cortical cells: Their developmental properties in normal and dark reared kittens. *J. Physiol.* (London), 1976, 255, 511–525.

Changeux, J. P., Courrege, P., & Danchin, A. A theory of the epigenesis of neuronal networks by selective stabilization of synapses. *Proc. Nat. Acad. Sci. USA*, 1973, *70*, No. 10, 2974–2978.

Cooper, L. N., Liberman, F., & Oja, E. A theory for the acquisition and loss of neuron specificity in visual cortex. *Biol. Cybernetics,* 1979, *33,* 9–28.

Creutzfeldt, O. D., Kuhnt, U., & Benevento, L. A. An intracellular analysis of visual cortical neurones to moving stimuli: Responses in a cooperative neuronal network. *Exp. Brain Res.,* 1974, *21,* 251.

Davis, T. L., & Sterling, P. Microcircuitry of cat visual cortex: Classification of neurons in layer IV of area 17, and identification of the patterns of lateral geniculate input. *J. Comp. Neurol.,* 1979, *188,* 599.

Fregnac, Y. *Cinetique de developpement du cortex visuel primaire chez le chat. Effets de la privation visuelle binoculaire et modele de maturation de la selective a l'orientation.* Doctoral thesis, Université René Descartes, Paris, 1978.

Fregnac, Y., & Imbert, M. Cinetique de developpement du cortex visuel. *J. Physiol.* (Paris), 1977, *6,* (Vol. 73).

Fregnac, Y., & Imbert, M. Early development of visual cortical cells in normal and dark-reared kittens: Relationship between orientation selectivity and ocular dominance. *J. Physiol.* (London), 1978, *278,* 27–44.

Hebb, D. O. *The organization of behavior.* New York: Wiley, 1949.

Hornung, J. P., & Garey, L. J. The thalamic projection to cat visual cortex: Ultrastructure of neurons identified by golgi impregnation or retrograde horseradish peroxidase transport. *Neuroscience,* 1981, *6,* 1053.

Hubel, D. H., & Wiesel, T. N. Receptive fields of single neurons in the cat striate cortex. *J. Physiol.* (London), 1959, *148,* 574–591.

Imbert, M., & Buisseret, Y. Receptive field characteristics and plastic properties of visual cortical cells in kittens reared with or without visual experience. *Exp. Brain Res.,* 1975, *22,* 2–36.

Kasamatsu, T., & Pettigrew, J. D. Depletion of brain catecholamines: Failure of ocular dominance shift after monocular occlusion in kittens. *Science,* 1976, *194,* 206–209.

Kasamatsu, T., & Pettigrew, J. D. Preservation of binocularity after monocular deprivation in the striate cortex of kittens treated with 6-hydroxydopamine. *J. Comp. Neurol.,* 1979, *185,* 139–162.

Kohonen, T. Associative memory: A system theoretic approach. Berlin: Springer–Verlag, 1977.

Kratz, K. E., & Spear, P. D. Effects of visual deprivation and alterations in binocular competition on responses of striate cortex neurons in the cat. *J. Comp. Neurol.,* 1976, *170,* 141.

Leventhal, A. G., & Hirsch, H. V. B. Effects of early experience upon orientation sensitivity and binocularity of neurons in visual cortex of cats. *Proc. Nat. Acad. Sci. USA,* 1977, *74,* No. 3, 1272–1276.

Leventhal, A. G., & Hirsch, H. V. B. Receptive field properties of different classes of neurons in visual cortex of normal and dark-reared cats. *J. Neurophysiol.,* 1980, *43,* 1111.

Nass, M. M., & Cooper, L. N. A theory for the development of feature detecting cells in visual cortex. *Biol. Cybernetics,* 1975, *19,* 1–18.

Perez, R., Glass, L., & Shlaer, R. J. Development of specificity in the cat visual cortex. *J. Math. Biol.,* 1975, *1,* 275.

Sillito, A. M. The contribution of inhibitory mechanisms to the receptive field properties of neurons in the cat's striate cortex. *J. Physiol.,* 1975, *250,* 304–330.

Von der Malsburg, C. Self-organization of orientation sensitive cells in the striate cortex. *Kybernetik,* 1973, *14,* 85.

Watkins, D. W., Wilson, J. R., & Sherman, S. M. Receptive field properties of neurons in binocular and monocular segments of striate cortex in cats raised with binocular lid suture. *J. Neurophysiol.,* 1978, *41,* 322.

Wiesel, T. N., & Hubel, D. H. Single-cell responses in striate cortex of kittens deprived of vision in one eye. *J. Neurophysiol.,* 1963, *26,* 1003–1017.

Wiesel, T. N., & Hubel, D. H. Comparisons of the effects of unilateral and bilateral eye closure on cortical unit responses in kittens. *J. Neurophysiol.,* 1965, *28,* 1029–1040.

10 Tuesday's Discussion

Pettigrew: Leon, I wanted to follow up on the question Jerry raised about whether there was any constraint on the final product in the sense that you might have just been bringing out a structure that was already there. I wasn't all that surprised about the results you got. Even if one takes the most radical empiricist point of view, the brain, the visual cortex is completely modifiable, and there's no innate specificity. Hebb has described that view and, for the sake of argument, you can take that point of view. But one still has to explain why it is that, when the cells eventually get their orientation specificities, neighboring cells have similar specificities, and when cells organize for ocular dominance, they do so in especially organized ways. That is, you have long linear domains with one eye and other long linear domains with the other eye. My question is: What special constraints are in your algorithm? There must be at least one, because you don't have an infinite array. That is, if you assume random interconnectivity, your matrix ends. It's got boundaries, so there is at least one spatial constraint.

Cooper: Perhaps I wasn't completely clear because I began by talking about the case where there was a large number of output cells, but then I switched to talking about the output of a single cell. Now, in order to give the results that I showed, we assumed no interaction between the cortical cells. In other words, a single cell can become selective or lose its selectivity without reference to any other cortical cell. However, there's nothing that prevents us from putting in cortical excitation or inhibition — we did that previously. It's just that you don't need those assumptions for the single-cell result. In order to get the orientation column and the gradual progression, there's no doubt that you're going to have to build in cortical–cortical interaction. Probably the kind of thing that will give you the lineup of the columns is some kind of excitation along the column, and the thing that does give you the rotation is inhibition between neighboring columns. We have run simulations; it sort of works. I think many people have gotten that result. But that was not mentioned in what I showed you because in this particular work we're not talking about the organization of the columns or the rotation. We're talking about the output of a single cell. I must add that it is not intuitively obvious what assumptions you have to make to come out with these single-cell results.

Pettigrew: I was most impressed by the fact that you came up with a device for adjusting the threshold; my experience with these kinds of models in the past has been that it's very difficult because the result is sort of brittle. For example, Von der Malsburg has done similar things. But if you try to replicate those results, you find that the numerical values which you have to plug in to get the result are extremely brittle.

Cooper: Yes, you're absolutely right. In fact, we went through that stage. We originally just put Θ_m and everything was very brittle, but on further thought it was obvious that there is no reason to put it in one place rather than another place. The most obvious thing seemed to be to attach it to some property of the cell.

Pettigrew: Would you like to speculate on what might be going on in the nerve cell that's moving the threshold up and down so far? It seems to me that is perhaps the most important prediction, rather than guessing what different conditions would do.

Crick: Well, it doesn't have to be very fast.

Cooper: No, it's not very fast. There are several times involved, and it's a rather slow process, actually. It depends on the average activity of the cell and can adjust relatively slowly; it's certainly not something that has to be done in milliseconds. I don't know what the actual times are, but that's a very interesting question to ask and one potentially capable of an experimental answer. What we really do is make the minimum number of assumptions in order to get a little structure. When you get to a stage where you have to make assumptions, you make them.

Pettigrew: A very strong prediction would be one about timing. I think that the results of the other predictions, such as what's going to happen when you do identical patterns to both eyes, will be less surprising.

Cooper: What does one get, by the way?

Pettigrew: You do get correlation between the two eyes. We found that in the planetarium experiment with the kittens. The only thing is that the cells you get are rather unusual.

Cooper: You got correlations between the two eyes?

Pettigrew: The cells, if they're selective, have similar selectivity in the two eyes. And even if they're nonselective, they're always on in one eye and on in the other. You don't get a cell which is off in one eye and on in the other. Mike Stryker has used tetrodotoxin to stop all spontaneous activity emanating from the eye. He then electrically stimulates the two optic nerves. In other words, he's got absolute control over the timing. What he doesn't have control over is the fact that the on and off cells are going to be active simultaneously.

Cooper: He also doesn't have control over the patterns that are put in. The patterns put into each eye will not be the same.

Pettigrew: Well, in a strict sense, he does because he's putting in a pattern that would never exist in the normal life of on and off cells.

Cooper: I'd have to think about that, but I suspect that he's doing overall electrical stimulation, and he's really not having the patterns coming into the two eyes.

Pettigrew: There's a terrific constraint there — you're going to have exactly synchronous activity of cells that normally would never be activated. Normally they'd be mutually inhibitory. If he does get cells which can be driven by electrical stimulation in both optic nerves, that will be a fulfillment of your prediction. It would also be a fulfillment of extreme radical empiricism.

Cooper: We have to be very careful about what a fulfillment of prediction turns out to be. Let me just ask you: Do you think that the determination of a certain time would be very significant in an experimental situation? What time is it that you're interested in?

Crick: There's a misunderstanding about the word "fast." You used the word "fast" in two senses. When he says "fast," he means to a higher power than 1. And then people take it to mean that it happens in a short time.

Cooper: When I say that the modification threshold, Θ_m, moves rapidly, I mean that it moves more rapidly than the average output of the cell. If the average output of the cell shifts, Θ_m shifts more. But whether it happens fast in time or slow in time is an independent question.

Pettigrew: It wouldn't depend on the cell, would it?

Cooper: The speed with which the process takes place does depend on the environment and on what's happening, but we've had to make no special assumptions about the speed. If I recall properly, one consequence is that learning is faster than unlearning, as Erkki Oja put it. In other words, the loss of information due to noise seems to go more slowly than the gain of information due to patterns. That seems to be built in by the nature of the system. But that's the only thing I can say about actual speed at the moment.

Pettigrew: Could I rephrase what you've said by saying that the mechanism for adjusting the threshold has to move faster than the mean level of activity?

Cooper: That's right.

Pettigrew: That is a considerable constraint in a cellular–biological context.

Cooper: I agree with you, and that's one of the things that has to be there.

Arbib: I'd like to address a question to Professor Kohonen. We have been playing with different variations on the Hebb synapse, and I think we've just seen a demonstration that a sort of mixture of Hebb and anti-Hebb seems to have certain virtues in setting up a stability analysis. But what strikes me very much is the fact that you set these synapses up in visual cortex. You hit them with certain patterns, and you end up with a bunch of orientation-tuned neurons. Now, Professor Kohonen started his talk with a list of something like seven different systems which he felt could be tuned by a common mechanism. They ranged all the way from laminar-associative memories, to temporally tuned networks, to novelty filters, and so on. This raises a question: What is it in the genetic setup of a system that determines what it will do? What is it that says, with a given synaptic rule, you will become a thing which tunes up line detectors? What is it that tunes you up to become a detector of temporal patterns? What is it that sets you up to become a novelty system?

Kohonen: If I understand him correctly, Dr. Pettigrew said in his paper that plasticity is a function of time, so that the α constant that I have in my equation could be a function of time. So, in the first place, for one set of neurons, you could have plasticity for, let's say, a few weeks. These neurons could be on a rather low level of the hierarchical system. When they are consolidated, they start acting like more specific detectors, and the higher level still has plasticity or starts to gain plasticity. And this plasticity, which is a function of time in different systems, can be controlled genetically by genetic order or development, which further could be influenced by various chemicals like hormones or any type of biochemical control.

Arbib: You might imagine the difference as being analogous to tuning in low-level detectors first and then tuning in higher-level macrodetectors. But what about the difference between things like spatial and temporal patterns or things like the difference between association and novelty detection?

Kohonen: For the storage and recall of temporal patterns, what you need extra is some feedback that is not internal to the network but more remote; so the type or structure of feedback paths would be different from the basic model. If you have a feedback through the thalamus or other parts, you have another type of system than if your feedback is by the collaterals. In the latter case, you don't have any significant delay in the feedback path. In the first case, you have a significant delay, which is higher than the temporal resolution between the signal patterns that come in.

Arbib: My final question is kind of a bridge between what you've been talking about and what Dr. Cooper was talking about. How is it that some cells know how to become simple and other cells know how to become complex? I don't think the models are addressing this, are they?

Cooper: There's no definite answer to that. Just let me give an illustration — I'm not saying this is the way it is — but if, for example, there's a cell in a column that is tied in, that can be excited by a large number of what we call simple cells that are more or less attuned to the same orientation, with little spread in their receptive field, then, by any of these rules, that would become a complex cell. Maybe you would like to add something to that, Wolf.

Singer: Well, I wanted to make a more general comment which ties into this problem. If these models are to make predictions about physiology, they have to take into account the huge amount of available data. A cortical neuron is a structure whose connectivity is to a large extent determined genetically, so the degrees of freedom a particular neuron has are largely determined by its position within the network and hence by its specific input–output connections. Thus, the question whether or not noncorrelated interocular input would give different receptive fields in the two eyes depends critically on whether the input stage has neurons with prespecified receptive field properties which serve as seeding grains for the subsequent organization of the functional architecture. If such is the case, even noncorrelated input is likely to give identical receptive field properties in both eyes. And there is evidence from cats that grew up with only one eye open but remained binocular that the receptive fields stay identical in the two eyes. Although noise was coming from one eye and structured activity from the other, the receptive field orientations were identical in the two eyes. This is to be expected if there are seeding grains right from the beginning that consist of a few prespecified neurons in Layer 4 that work as a crystallization point for the subsequent up positional of columnar development systems.

Cooper: This is one of the reasons I tried to be very cautious about making predictions. We are talking about a general mechanism; if you want to make predictions, you have to look at the particular system and put in relevant details.

Daniels: I want to make a comment about what I see as an assumption of all three presentations this morning — that nerve cells are capable of dealing with their inputs only with an algebraic summation operation, and that a consequence of this is that nerve cells don't really need dendrites, that synapses large and small can land right on the cell body, and that, from that point of view, the synapse is the only good, modifiable part of the surface. But if dendrites are enforcers of a distributive law for two operations, then a different site for plasticity can be seen, I think. That would be the tree trunk, where the information converges right at the cell bodies. It crosses through dendritic bifurcations, say, all in the left eye, or the primed eye input. Then, when information has to pass through the trunk on the way to the cell body, an increase or a decrease in the diameter of that trunk would change the influence of that eye on the output response. That trunk is really right next to the cell body, and you don't have worries about dendrites and synapses being very far from the cell body that's producing the output response. I'd like to hear all three comment on what I see as that assumption of "only one kind of operation" in the calculation ability of a neuron model.

Cooper: My answer is that when I say "synapse," it's a manner of speaking. The reason you say the change is at the synapse is because it's a common expression that is used, but all you really want is a change between the input signal coming from the axon and the potential that finally arrives at the axon hillock. If that occurs at the synapse, fine. If it occurs in the trunk, fine. It could occur in a group of synapses. It makes no difference logically if it occurs at the actual synapse. It's really just a manner of speaking.

Crick: I think you're evading the question because the point is that there are a lot of different synapses on one dendrite. He's saying that if you alter the diameter of a dendritic region you alter the weights of all the synapses there.

Cooper: I didn't realize the full implication of what you were saying. You must preserve the information coming from cells on the input side to cells on the output side. If you muddle them up in one dendrite, then things would not work.

Kohonen: This problem has been discussed before, although not at this conference. The first thing to realize is that there are different choices for the basic units of the network. It can be a group of neurons like an aggregate in a column, or it can be a part of a neuron, for instance, one branch in a giant neuron. There are neurons which can even trigger at the branches. It is only an arbitrary choice that we take one uniform unit. We could have a mixture of units with various sizes, with a distribution that is noncorrelated with the signals. It doesn't make a big difference. If I understand correctly, your question is "Do the synapses play a different role if they are located far out in the apical dendrites or at the shaft or at the synapses at one branch of the shaft?" Well, I completely agree that there would be a difference, but whether this is significant from the point of view of modeling is another question; namely, if the interconnections are made at least quasi-random. So, if the interconnections hit one or another branch of the shaft in a completely random fashion, there will be no correlation between the different sensitivities, or plasticities of the synapses. In the final evaluation of the output, we have random weights for different synapses, but there is a law of ergodicity in statistics that could be applied here. We can replace the distribution of plasticities by an average value. The variance in plasticities only adds an extra component of noise.

Crick: But you have to be careful about contrasting the neuron as a unit and the dendrite as a unit because it's only the cell that fires.

Sherman: That's not necessarily true. There can be local dendro–dendritic connections, and there are lots of these.

Crick: In the cortex?

Sherman: Everywhere. They're found everywhere.

Crick: In the neocortex?

Sherman: I don't know the answer to that. Certainly, they're there in the thalamus.

Crick: I know, but they're not necessarily in the neocortex.

Sherman: No one's looked for them there; that may be why they have not been found there.

Cowan: I want to ask Gordon Shepherd whether there are dendro–dendritic synapses in the neocortex.

Shepherd: Well, I think the situation might be likened to the situation in basal ganglia or in substantia nigra 5 or 6 years ago. At that time, a similar statement could have been made that there were no synapses observed in those structures between dendrites. Now that situation has been radically altered, and there's a great deal of interest in those kinds of interactions.

Crick: That's by analogy, but what's the answer to the question?

Shepherd: The answer really goes back to what Murray said, and that is that I think the cortex is the most difficult area in which to address that question for neuroanatomy. I don't think that comparable work has been done in that structure, though it's been done in other areas.

Crick: But I'm mildly surprised that they haven't seen them since everybody's been interested in this for the last five or ten years. I won't say they aren't there at all, but I doubt that they're there in large quantities.

Sherman: Well, it's not a trivial problem. It's always been assumed that if you see a synapse, it comes from an axon. But to demonstrate where it comes from requires serial section, and you have to reconstruct the whole cell. Techniques to do that are only now becoming readily available. So failure to demonstrate it at this point may not mean a great deal.

Shepherd: There's another thing: It's clear that interactions between neurons do not occur just at morphological specializations which we call synaptic junctions. I think that's becoming quite clear to anyone working with peptides or molecules of that nature. So I would assume it would be unwise to state that there aren't interactions between dendrites that might have some functional significance. The other thing to say is that there must be an enormous amount of activity within a given neuronal dendritic tree which is subthreshold, so that to judge what's going on in a neuron simply by the impulse output at the cell body is to take a very limited perspective.

Crick: If you've got five dendrites on a cell and one axon, I don't deny there may be small interactive effects between dendrites – those are second-order effects. We have those in molecular biology and they confuse things all the time. I don't believe they're important here. The point is, when the axon fires, how does it know which dendrite it came from? I think the major effects are due to the axons. And therefore I think these other effects are just producing complications where we have enough difficulties already. I don't believe they are going to turn out to be really important in the end.

Cooper: Just a comment on that. I think it should be said that, for most of this theoretical work, the use of the word "synapse" as the site at which modification occurs is a matter of convenience. What one really should say is that certain input–output relations hold and that they could be at what is known as a synapse, or they could be at a broader level; they could involve a number of synapses. It's obvious that we're not necessarily talking about a single connection. It's a very complex system, and what we're really saying is that certain subsystems, whatever they are, have properties of the type that have been described.

Shepherd: We shouldn't neglect the fact that all synapses or all junctions or all interconnections, however you want to conceive of them, are not equal, that the synapses on a spine are likely to have radically different properties from the synapses on a cell body. Although they may not be relevant to the discussion at this point, it's certainly going to be relevant at the next stage.

Crick: Yes, but something that is slurred over in discussing weights is that the weights don't have a time attached to them. In their treatment, they really use a digital approach. The weight is either there or it isn't. No allowance is made for time effects. If you took just a simple model where all synapses were the same and differed only in position, then you would think that any activation near the soma or the base of the dendrite would give you a short, sharp potential change at the axon hillock, and anything further away would give you a smaller, longer change. You're making, I think, an additional point—that they can be different in still other ways. I would agree because we know in fact that the synapses on most of the cell bodies in the cortex are inhibitory, so they are Type 2 not Type 1.

Shepherd: I'm not sure I understand all the degrees of freedom you're referring to in the way synapses can control neural output, but let me just mention one. You may already have made the point, but it's this: We may think of a synapse far out on a dendrite as being involved in only very slow modulation vis-à-vis the axonal output. But what if there's a site of active impulse generation out on the dendrite? Then it can gate something that's very rapid.

Crick: Well, of course, it's a question of whether dendrites are passive or active or semiactive. Unfortunately, we are not addressing that, but I agree with you that's what we want to know.

Shepherd: Then it goes back to the fact that a neuron is not one simple blob.

Crick: What do you mean by that?

Shepherd: It's not one simple summing site. It's not one simple input–output device.

Crick: What is it then?

Shepherd: It's a multiple input–output device, a distributive input–output device.

Singer: A question arises from your assumption that there's also a negative Hebb region which would switch off certain synapses when the postsynaptic response is available but does not reach consolidation threshold at the receptive site. One needs a mechanism that prevents a neuron which receives thousands of inputs from disconnecting all these inputs in favor of one input that is doing just the Hebb modification. I think it calls for local Hebbian mechanisms that are restricted to particular sites on dendrites. In that case, one wouldn't like to have the actual potential of the cell really be the postsynaptic signal. In any case, it's very unlikely that postsynaptic spikes reach threshold because they are damped substantially by the dendrites. An action potential is a very fast, biphasic event, that is unlikely to invade dendrites without substantial decrement and deformation. So I think that one might as well regard the required postsynaptic response as consisting of local dendritic responses, circumscribed potential changes within restricted postsynaptic compartments. There may be one type of modification going on in one part of the dendrite and another type in another part. The basal dendrite may not be participating in any adaptive changes while modifications occur at the apical dendrite.

Cooper: That is of course possible. Another, even simpler possibility is that some of the synaptic contacts are just not marked by them, and others are.

Crick: You have to state which ones and where they are; you have to state whether they're nearer the soma or something like that.

Cooper: We have to say that eventually, I agree.

Crick: There are rules about what types of synapse are on the soma and what are not.

Kohonen: We were talking about the simplest paradigm in this case. It is up to you how much complexity you want of a model. If you want different plasticity for every synapse, depending on the distance from the soma, that is all right. There can be synapses with different transmitters and different plasticity. There can be interaction between nearby synapses in the plasticity law. In fact, we have analyzed these cases. The only thing is that the formulas become more and more complicated. Instead of having scalar plasticity constants, we then have matrix plasticity constants, and this makes all these cases analyzable, although we have never published the results.

Edelman: I'd like to ask Dr. Anderson and Dr. Kohonen a question about these correlation matrices. I'd like to know how sensitive they are to variations in the precision of the terms. If you get large changes or even small changes in the individual terms over some time, will you get the same result or will it rapidly degrade? Since your result depends upon both a cross product and other terms, what about this fluctuation?

Anderson: As a general rule, all these correlation matrix systems are very noise resistant. In fact, in some cases, they're optimally noise resistant, in at least a mean square sense. This has to do with the way they're constructed. A lot of similar techniques are used in communication theory to optimally extract signals in radar systems.

Edelman: I'm asking the question because, if it were otherwise, you'd have to have rather precise values.

Anderson: The simulations were very precise; they worked quite well with a lot of noise in the system. This is something we've checked.

Kohonen: In an early publication from 1969 I made an analysis of this. For instance, if you destroy randomly a part of the correlation matrix, you introduce only a little more noise into the output. So you can destroy half of the memory elements without significant degradation of recall.

Edelman: But suppose every term in the matrix varies by ± 10%?

Anderson: If it has Gaussian variation, that has very little effect. In a series of simulations by Chris Wood that appeared in *Psychological Review,* he destroyed various parts of the matrix and various input cells and output cells. It degrades in what's called a graceful degradation.

Kohonen: It is also possible to have binary memory elements, not even continuous in value. The recall accuracy is not much worse than if you evaluate the memory elements by a ten-digit accuracy.

Edelman: But if that's the case, to maintain the same accuracy, your system has to get larger and larger.

Kohonen: You have usually plenty of input neurons. The dimensionality of the input might be as high as 10^8 neurons. When you sum up that many terms, you can easily discretize each one into binary classes without introducing particularly great errors in summation.

Anderson: Theoretically, and in terms of pure simulations, these models are very resistant to noise and to damage. This actually shows up in the simulations.

Edelman: But do they have finite capacities.

Anderson: Yes, they have finite capacities.

Kohonen: If you have a class of representations, you can form an average over them. You can form clusters. In that case, the models have an infinite capacity.

Edelman: I don't agree with that. Any finite-state machine whatsoever has a finite memory capacity.

Kohonen: The state of these systems values, at least the expectation values, can be continuous.

Edelman: They use finite hardware.

Anderson: It depends on how you use these systems. In many cases you want them not to have too many states. For example, you may want to classify things into categories or into particular types; you may want to know whether a certain letter is an *A* or a *B* or a *C,* for example, even though it may appear in degraded form. This is a typical psychologically oriented task.

Elbaum: Is it really important whether the system has finite or infinite capacity, as long as the capacity exceeds by a large factor any conceivable need?

Edelman: Well, it's theoretically interesting.

Arbib: First a comment and then a question. The comment is this: I think that it's very important to understand what a particular mechanism can do and to be able to study it in isolation. It is important that we build up a vocabulary of mechanisms so that, when we're faced with a new problem, we can try to combine elegantly what we know to address that problem. I get a little uncomfortable when I hear from a few people what I call experimental imperialism, which is that a theory is not of any value unless it addresses all the experimental data. It would seem to me that an analogous approach would be for those of you who study monkeys to reject any work by an aplysiologist unless it could be shown that the circuit was in fact an exact replica of one that occurred in a mammalian form.

Poggio: Oh, we do. We do. [laughter]

Arbib: As long as your objection is in that spirit, as long as you think of us as being another form of spineless neuroscientists, then that's all right. And now the question: Dr. Anderson confessed that he's been speaking to psychologists — we deserve an explanation. It seems to me that the explanation can be of two different kinds. One is to say that there are interesting problems and experiments in learning theory, in animal learning, and so on, that he can explain. I suspect that when he says that he can now explain these things, he does not claim that the elements in his networks are actually neurons, but perhaps correspond to sort of abstract clumps in the brain, but no more. On the other hand, he might wish to say more strongly that, from his acquaintance with the psychologists, he can think of new experiments that would challenge the people in neuroplasticity. Perhaps you can address both those issues.

Anderson: I wish I could be that concrete. I would love to come up with experiments that I really felt could be testable at the neurophysiological level at this time. I think one clearly has in these distributive models an interesting class of models from a psychological point of view. One of the things that's striking about these models is that retrieval is a very short process. A distributive system lets you know whether something is stored or not stored in essentially one computational step. So you have a very rapid means of retrieving information from a very large data base. And this appears to be true of some aspects of human memory, in that you can tell with a very quick computation whether or not a word has been seen before. There are a lot of qualitative comments of that kind that one can look into in more detail. I've actually fitted some of these models to some of this data. Unfortunately, you're quite right — we can't say, "Okay, the fact that you've got neurons of a particular kind in cortex leads you to a particular kind of model," but certainly distributive models along the lines I've presented do give a pretty good account of themselves, explaining a lot of psychological data in a qualitative way. And they can be made quite precise, in that they can fit the psychological data in the sense of fitting reaction-time curves and that kind of thing. The connection is not as tight as one would like, but the hope is that it can be and will be made.

Cowan: Since Jim's been talking with psychologists, I wanted to ask him exactly how the associative memory system relates to all the things that psychologists do on human memory. Are you talking about short-term memory, or episodic memory, or recognition memory, or syntactic memory? What predictive value has the correlation memory system with regard to that? I hear people who say, "Well, real memory has nothing whatsoever to do with these correlation systems. It all has to do with cognitive maps—the Tolman theory rather than all this stuff." They say that a lot of it is so context dependent that, unless you can get the context in, it doesn't mean anything.

Anderson: I'm not quite sure how to answer that. It is true that human memory in a cognitive sense is an immensely difficult thing. There are a few specific experiments—for example, some of the visual-search experiments and the list-scanning experiments—where you can make very precise models which incorporate some of these distributive notions and which actually work. But explaining the whole range of human memory with these models is extremely difficult.

Cowan: But which range of human memory are these models aimed at? What psychological phenomena do they really address?

Anderson: The specific example that we've looked at most carefully is the Sternberg list-scanning experiments, where we had a quite precise model based on some of these principles, a model that can fit the data as well or better than anybody else's model, if you talk about curve fitting. I'm not sure how valid that is. We all know that it's very easy to make models fit data. The more interesting thing has to do with general patterns of response. For example, in the brain-in-a-box model, one tends to extract the most significant information first and the least significant last. We have time courses of that kind that are at least in qualitative agreement. One sees categorization effects that are very powerful.

Cowan: Could you say anything about Shepard's experiments?

Anderson: The mental rotation experiments? Those are very intriguing. I think that we may be looking there at a case of a special-purpose black box that our correlation models may say nothing to. I think some of the other effects that one sees in semantic memory—word retrieval, some aspects of semantic retrieval, visual memory, for example—may be explainable by correlation effects with nonlinearities.

Cowan: Don't you think that everything in the nervous system is made up of special-purpose black boxes?

Anderson: No, I wouldn't say that.

Liberman: Some of the experiments in speech perception get very much to the point of how constructive these models are. Any constructivist model will extract signals only if there are parameters in the physical signal that will partition the signal. The whole notion of the Haskins speech-perception theory with two-formant patterns ([ba], [da], [ga]) is that there are no attributes of the signal that will partition this. Now, if these experiments with 13-week-old infants can be pushed back toward birth and if neonates partition the speech sounds into categories, then we have to assume special hardware adapted, probably through natural selection, to these sounds.

Anderson: In fact, one of our models is specifically applied to some of these categorization phenomena in speech, and they at least reproduce the qualitative aspects of behavior.

Liberman: But you can't get a two-formant pattern that way. That's really the crucial question; there is no parameter in the physical signal that will allow you to specify the templates.

Anderson: Not necessarily. That has to do with how these algorithms work.

Kučera: But Stevens and Blumstein argue differently, Phil.

Liberman: But if you go back to the two-formant pattern, it doesn't work.

Kohonen: I think that much of this discussion is along the lines of what I call scientific voodoo: you make a sacrificial model of your opponent and then you punch him. The whole brain is not a matter of mathematics. We had a stimulating discussion a year and a half ago at another conference of this type. The general notion of the modelers was that we should compare these models, model matrices, with chips of computers, and not with the computers themselves. And the organization, which can be partly genetic, takes care of much of this hierarchical information processing. But the important thing to realize is that the elements can have adaptive properties. Now it is very easy to stifle a discussion by saying that we are then not modeling the brain. By the way, we can also handle semantic data and other relational structures with laminar models. Instead of having pictoral, iconic patterns, your pattern is then composed of different subfields where you have different attributes.

Edelman: Phil, you provoked me, but I'm not sure I understood what you said about formant patterns in very young infants.

Liberman: Yes. There are experiments that are now classic, the first one by Peter Eimas. Thirteen-week old infants will partition synthetic speech signals for the syllables [ba], [da], and [ga] using two-formant patterns. In other words, these two-formant patterns represent the classic dimension of place of articulation for human languages — labials, dentals, and velars.

Kučera: The partition of a continuum into binary discrete locations.

Liberman: I should add that these are impoverished signals — there is no direct physical property in these signals. You have to posit that these patterns are inside the organism in order to get this partitioning.

Edelman: You mean that nobody has yet produced an algorithm.

Liberman: That's impossible.

Edelman: You are saying that it's innate, innate in that there's some special structure that's already built in.

Kučera: But, curiously, not only for humans, because chinchillas have the same mechanism.

Liberman: The speech signal's very nice in that, if you give a fully specified signal with the bursts in all formants, you can derive a physical parameter that will give you invariant locations.

Kučera: Maybe. For initial position.

Liberman: But if you take these simplified signals, people will again partition them in the same places. Now, for adults, you can say, "Well, perhaps a machine of the sort described today would work" — they might have initially learned the full pattern and they still respond to a small part of it.

Edelman: You're implying that the infants had no prior experience of this kind in a training phase.

Liberman: The crucial experiment will be to push this down toward birth. If the infant still responds in this way, it would provide evidence for special hardware. It's interesting because that's the only evidence that Chomsky has ever come up with for an innate mechanism. No innate mechanisms have ever been demonstrated for syntax.

Reeke: I wanted to return to the point about the various possible mechanisms of synaptic modification. Each of the three speakers, I think, emphasized that the exact rule used can have a large effect on the type of dynamic behavior the system gives. And yet in the end each speaker, I think, talked about only one such rule. I would like to ask anyone who could answer what other rules were tried and, in particular, what part of the rule has to do with the interesting dynamic response of the system and what parts had to be put in just to obtain stability. Since stability can be obtained in a neural network, I should think there would be various other mechanisms such as overall levels of certain chemicals, or what have you. If you obtain stability some other way, you will have more freedom in choosing your modification rules. Have any of these gentlemen explored other rules?

Kohonen: I gave a paper which solved the problems by assuming heterosynaptic facilitation and not Hebbian synapses. There have been some attempts to model the adaptive phenomena without the Hebbian rule, for instance, the Von der Malsburg paper. It had a linear superposition of presynaptic signals and a threshold. The problem is that such a model is rather sensitive to parameter values. You had to have very accurate parameters in order for it to operate. The correlation matrix or Hebbian-type laws, on the other hand, are very insensitive to parameters.

Cooper: In what we did, you need the negative slope at the origin, the positive slopes at the crossover, and the variation of the crossover going faster (not in time) than the average activity of the cell in order to get agreement with the various experiments I showed. If you abandon any one of these, you won't get agreement.

Reeke: Is that a proved theorem or an empirical result?

Edelman: He's constructed a system which is bistable.

Cooper: It's a consequence of the assumptions. We have some analytic results and have run computer simulations that verify all of these points.

McIlwain: There's another proved theorem, and that is that the cerebrum will function only so long.

11 A Model of Cortical Associative Memory

Teuvo Kohonen and Erkki Oja
Helsinki University of Technology

Pekka Lehtiö
University of Helsinki

The modeling approach to associative memory discussed in this chapter derives from more general efforts to outline the mechanisms of memory in physical systems, especially when these mechanisms are embodied in a large collection of interacting elements. However, when contrasted with many other more mathematical or universal modeling approaches, our present aim is to relate this idea directly to a concrete cortical structure.

The basic associative memory operation is selective recall of a stored signal pattern by a key stimulus. The idea that this function is based on some kind of "holographic" principle has been widely discussed in theoretical neuroscience. The key feature by virtue of which such a principle has been adopted by many neuroscientists is that memory traces representing a certain piece of information are distributed all over the neural tissue. Optical holography as such, however, is not a good formalism for these effects because it relies on signal transformations very difficult to implement by the neural structures. Therefore it has become important to study alternative implementations of distributed memory mechanisms, in order to single out reasonable candidates to serve as models of distributed neural memory.

The study of associative memory necessarily leads also to discussion of more general neural information processing. Mechanisms for analysis of features or patterns contained in neural signals are sometimes seen to form the common conceptual basis for neuroanatomy, neurophysiology, and psychology (Leibovic, 1969). There are some interesting theoretical thoughts about these problems (e.g., the series of publications by H. B. Barlow leading to his neuron doctrine for perceptual psychology [Barlow, 1972] and the work of Warren McCulloch, 1965). Far more common, however, has been the objection that the problems of specific information processing should be postponed until more is known about the structure and function of the neural network.

For system theorists the problems of signal processing and adaptive mechanisms have always been natural objectives of theoretical study that have led, moreover, to very practical applications in technology. But this research has also resulted in knowledge of powerful organizational principles and functional characteristics that are transferable to neural circuits and networks, too. Based on such concepts it is possible to develop physical system models of associative memory that are useful in defining information-processing principles to clarify, for instance, how information is represented in networks or which stages of transformations signal patterns may undergo.

Traditional neuroanatomy and neurophysiology have approached the brain trying to discover *specific* circuits or functions. There has been a lack of paradigms that would describe *collective* phenomena. One objective in system theory has therefore been to describe the latter in pure or idealized form, even though real phenomena are usually mixtures, and there might exist a seeming discrepancy between theory and experiments for this reason. However, it has been considered extremely important to be able to devise new *working* and *quantitatively justified paradigms.* For instance, a model of memory must possess a storage for a great number of activity patterns, not just for one or two learned functions.

When dealing with a complicated system like the cortical network, one must be aware of the necessity of making certain simplifying assumptions in its modeling: first, one must limit oneself to a *small* number of general nonquantitative hypotheses that contain the essence of the model; and second, one must specify the consequences of these hypotheses at a level detailed and quantitative enough for mathematical analysis and computer simulations. In making these latter type of assumptions, there may exist alternative ways, all fitting within the general model framework and all producing essentially similar results. Therefore it becomes imperative to include only such features in the model that make it *really work* in the desired way (i.e., with regard to capacity, stability, etc.).

In models of *associative memory* relating to the cortical network, the crucial hypotheses must concern the learning and recollection mechanisms and the role of different neural units and connections in these processes. It seems nowadays generally accepted among neurophysiologists that synaptic changes in the connections between cortical neurons underlie memory and learning. However, an even more important step is to realize that it is not sufficient to find sensitizable or habituating *channels* but to explain what mechanisms make it possible to *selectively* impress memory traces and to read them fast and reliably, relating to specific input. To achieve this, every unit capable of storing a memory trace ought to have *at least two types of input control*: one for *data* to be stored, one for *addressing* or reading this data. Some recent experimental evidence seems to point to synaptic modification that fulfills these requirements (Levy, this volume; Rauschecker & Singer, 1979).

Another basic hypothesis concerns the concept of *distributed* memory. The CNS is not a collection of independent units but a highly interactive system. It seems that memory is spatially distributed in the cortical network. In order that this be possible, the memory traces must be encoded in a very *collective* way. Also, a *recollection* from memory cannot merely be represented by the activity of a separate neuron or other small information-processing unit, but as a collection of simultaneous activities, forming *spatial and temporal patterns,* and involving a considerable part of the neurons in the memory network. This is only possible if there exists between the neural units a dense network of *long-range interactions* that, because of the speed of recollection and the stability of the spatial patterns, would be expected to be essentially monosynaptic. It is interesting to note that the long-range, recurrent, mostly subcortical lateral connections of the cortical pyramidal neurons offer an anatomical basis for exactly such a system of interconnectivities (Braitenberg, 1978). There may exist similar intracortical connections through the neuropil.

In the following section we try to build a model of cortical associative memory along these lines.

LATERAL SPREADING OF EXCITATION IN THE CORTICAL NETWORK

To elucidate the role of different neural connectivities of the mammalian neocortex in memory functions, we refer to Fig. 11.1, which presents the well-known local spreading of excitation and inhibition around an arbitrary point of activity. The figure defines only the *lateral* spread; the correlation of activities in any given *vertical* penetration of the cortex is usually high enough to warrant the approximation of the distribution as essentially two-dimensional. For reasons of symmetry, this has been depicted in terms of one spatial coordinate only in the figure.

The short-range excitatory and inhibitory interactions in Fig. 11.1 are strictly distance dependent. Both are mediated by short intracortical axon collaterals of the pyramidal neurons as well as by various interneurons. The short-range excitatory connections reach laterally to a distance of about 50 to 100 μm (in primates), whereas the short-range inhibitory connections, primarily mediated through interneurons, extend to about 300 to 500 μm with a distribution strongly dependent on distance. This short-range connectivity

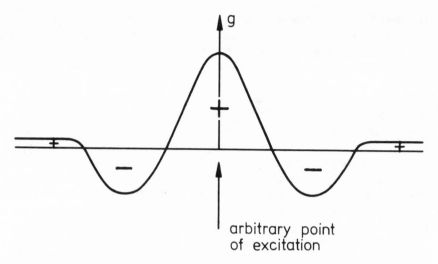

FIG. 11.1   Lateral spread of excitation and inhibition around an arbitrary point of activity in the cortex. This is the kernel function *g* used in Equation 1. *Plus sign:* excitation. *Minus sign:* inhibition.

has an important function in local signal processing like forming activity clusters, feature extraction, and signal transformations.

The inhibitory penumbra is again enclosed in a surround of weaker excitation. It does not seem to be experimentally verified how far this long-range excitatory interaction may spread; some authors hold a view that it is essentially independent of distance from the reference point of activity (Braitenberg, 1978). We now come to a crucial hypothesis in the present model of cortical distributed memory: we take the view that *the memory traces that are responsible for the associative memory function are located in the excitatory monosynaptic cortico–cortical connections.*

It has been pointed out by many neuroscientists (Creutzfeldt, 1976; Szentágothai, 1978) that the distribution of local structures (cell types and short-range interconnectivities) of the mammalian neocortex is strikingly uniform in the lateral direction over many different areas. This observation should be contrasted with a neurophysiological view according to which many areas of the cortex are functionally divided or organized into almost identical, vertically cylindrical units named "columns" (Hubel & Wiesel, 1974; Mountcastle, 1957). Functional columns with sharp borders can be found, for example, in primary sensory areas where, with a dimension of .5 to 1 mm, they seem to be organized around specific afferent signals. Signal activities within a column, especially between its principal neurons, seem to be highly correlated.

Nonetheless there prevails a certain degree of disagreement concerning the nature (for a review, see Towe, 1975) and general role of such "columns" in neurophysiology. The existence of such units in some primary sensory areas has been verified in the case of separate sensory organs projecting onto the same local area of cortex, notably in the case of ocular dominance columns or slabs in the primary visual cortex of some animals (Hubel & Wiesel, 1974) as well as in the somatosensory cortex (Mountcastle, 1957). In this case the roughly periodic division of the cortical sheet into columns is necessary to preserve the topological organization.

We now point out that, without committing oneself to any theories regarding the role of columns, it follows from the local short-range excitatory and inhibitory connectivity already discussed that the triggering activity of the cortex has a natural tendency to become *clustered* into cylindrical foci of the same dimension as that of the columns. To show this system-theoretically, consider a two-dimensional plate that shall represent the cortical cell mass in an ultimately simplified physical constitution (Fig. 11.2).

Denote the momentary signal activity (corresponding to some averaged triggering frequency) over the plate by a function $u = u(x, y, t)$, where x and y are the lateral spatial coordinates of a point, and t is the time parameter. If the cells, due to local interactions, integrate the activities of afferent excitation $f = f(x, y, t)$ as well as that of recurrent feedback from nearby cells, as defined by the excitability function $g(x, y)$ depicted in Fig. 11.1, then the time behavior of $u(x, y, t)$ is described by a system equation of the type

$$u(x, y, t) = \sigma[f + \iint g(r, s)u(x - r, y - s, t - \Delta t)drds]. \tag{1}$$

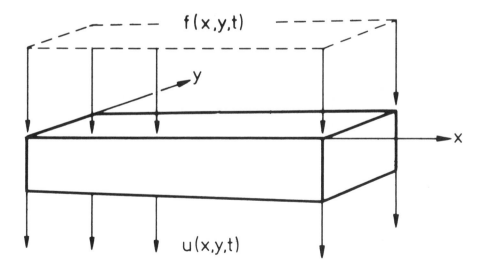

FIG. 11.2   Schematic view of the cortical cell mass shown as a two-dimensional plate. $f(x, y, t)$: the afferent excitation that is a function of the two spatial coordinates x and y and time t. $u(x, y, t)$: the efferent signal activity over the plate. The interconnectivity within cortex is not shown.

There $\sigma[\cdot]$ denotes a function that takes care of nonlinearities (triggering limits) and Δt is a time delay due to lateral feedback. A computer simulation, shown in Fig. 11.3, demonstrates qualitatively how a primary input distribution of activity (with two very different initial humps, shown shaded) develops in time according to Equation 1. In this simulation $\sigma[\cdot]$ was simply a piecewise linear function confined between two triggering limits at $u = 0$ and $u = u_{max}$.

In the following modeling approach we assume that the signal activity distributions over the cortex can be represented by clusters of the aforementioned type, without considering whether these coincide with possible columns or not. The intensities of the clusters form mosaiclike patterns over the cortex, and it is a collection of such spatial patterns that we are storing and retrieving in computer simulations of distributed memory models.

Notice that as long as $\sigma[\cdot]$ is a linear function without saturation limits, u follows f linearly. Another fact discernible from Fig. 11.3 is that the width of the cluster may depend on f. In modeling approaches, even if activity clustering takes place as in this model, proportionality of responses to input is a good approximation and is utilized further in the following section.

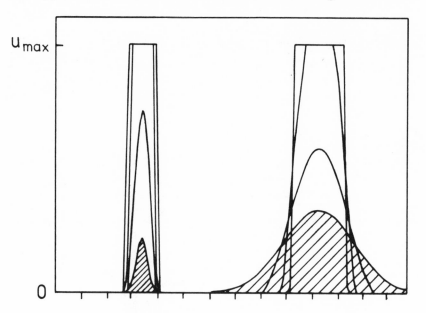

FIG. 11.3   Time development of local activity due to the short-range excitatory and inhibitory connections. *Lowest curve:* the initial activity, showing two humps. *Uppermost curve:* the stabilized activity resulting from Equation 1, showing clustering of activity. In the simulation, $g(r, s)$ had approximately the form shown in Fig. 11.1, with the width of the central excitatory region corresponding to one unit on the abscissa of Fig. 11.3, and σ was a linear function with saturation at 0 and u_{max}.

THE CORTICAL NETWORK AS AN ADAPTIVE SPATIAL FILTER

We have pointed out earlier in several discussions (see Kohonen, 1977) that the associative memory function of the brain is implementable without any principles resembling those of computer memories, if a neural network operates as an *adaptive filter.* Such a filter must comprise the following functions: (1) the pattern of simultaneous signal activities in a set of afferent axons is transformed into another pattern of simultaneous signal activities in another set of efferent axons. This transformation (in the frequency domain) need not be linear, although many times, at least when referring to statistical averages, it can be approximated by a linear *transfer function;* (2) the parameters of the transfer function are at all times adaptively changed due to the transmitted signals. In this way the responses not only depend on present input information but also on all earlier inputs. A crucial feature in such a memory principle must be that the filter selectively produces similar responses to similar inputs.

The possibility for existence of filters of the aforementioned type is demonstrated in this work. This model does not presuppose any complicated addressing, storage, and reading mechanisms like those stipulated by most alternative explanations of biological memory.

As stated previously, any adaptive changes in the signal transfer function of a neural network are primarily of synaptic origin. The Hebbian law, which has enjoyed an almost doctrinal status among modelers, has frequently been used to describe these changes; only recently (e.g., at this symposium) some experimental evidence for a law of this type has been brought forth.

The essence of the Hebbian law or hypothesis is that for any changes in the synaptic efficacy there must be present *both* a presynaptic *and* a postsynaptic factor; these factors are proportional to the triggering frequencies of presynaptic and postsynaptic neurons, respectively. There seems to be some controversy, however, concerning the exact way in which these factors should be taken into account. Some models even neglect the postsynaptic factor altogether, whereas others express the law for differential signals only.

The original Hebbian hypothesis (Hebb, 1949) is unsatisfactory as a process hypothesis at least for the following reasons: (1) it involves changes of efficacy in one direction only, which very soon leads out of the control range of variable parameters; (2) it does not provide any means for referring to a stable (idle) state at which no changes should occur in spite of ongoing background activity; and (3) to change the efficacy, the control factors (e.g., chemicals) ought to be synthesized very quickly within the cell.

For the aforementioned reasons we argue that a much more natural way of expressing the synaptic plasticity law, thereby taking into account both the presynaptic and the postsynaptic factor, is to assume that *the sum of synaptic efficacies within a cell is approximately constant,* at least over a short period (seconds), and *all significant short-term changes in relative efficacies of synapses must be due to redistribution in the cell of a postsynaptic factor that determines these efficacies.* A possible candidate for such a factor is the concentration of chemical receptor proteins at the postsynaptic membrane; nonetheless it is not necessary to commit oneself to this particular hypothesis. What seems to be essential is that the efficacy of a synapse μ be describable by a process of the type (Kohonen, 1977)

$$\frac{d\mu}{dt} = \alpha(\xi - \xi_b)\eta \tag{2}$$

where ξ is a presynaptic input (or triggering frequency of the presynaptic neuron), ξ_b is an effective background value, η is the postsynaptic triggering frequency, and α is a proportionality constant (that defines the degree of plasticity of this particular synapse).

In order to understand this law better, we might also describe the partition of such a factor between two nearby synapses with efficacies μ_1 and μ_2, and presynaptic inputs ξ_1 and ξ_2, respectively.

$$\frac{d\mu_1}{dt} = \alpha(\xi_1 - \xi_2)\eta$$

$$\frac{d\mu_2}{dt} = \alpha(\xi_2 - \xi_1)\eta \tag{3}$$

At uniform input $\xi_1 = \xi_2$, there will be no changes in either efficacy.

Now we are ready to set up the model of signal transformation in an *adaptive laminar network model* of cortex. Consider Fig. 11.4, which depicts an array of hypothetical principal neurons, each symbol possibly representing a large group of real neurons. Such a group may more accurately correspond to a column or an activity cluster. These elements form a two-dimensional, laminar array.

Each element (with label i) receives a primary input signal φ_i, as well as *long-range lateral feedback* from the outputs η_j of a large number of other elements in the same array. Local feedback of the type of Fig. 11.1 is now neglected, as it already caused the clustering of activity. Moreover, when we are now concentrating on the analysis of long-term effects, in such an extended time scale we might better regard φ_i, not as the primary input itself but as some kind of amplified and averaged activity referring to a "cluster," as in Fig. 11.3. Every η_i is assumed to depend on the other activities according to a law

$$\eta_i = F(\varphi_i + \sum_{j \in S_i} \mu_{ij}\eta_j) \tag{4}$$

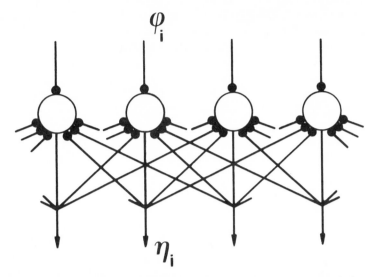

FIG. 11.4   Schematic presentation of the laminar network model. Each large circle represents a group of neurons whose activities are clustered due to the short-range interconnections, not shown in the figure. The feedback lines indicate long-range excitatory interconnections between the groups, which may reach any points in the network. φ_i: the afferent activity which is input to group i. η_i: the efferent activity of group i, which is fed back to a large number of other elements of the same network.

where $F(\cdot)$ is some (possibly nonlinear) function of its argument. The summation range S_i refers to a subset of elements j, which have a feedback connection to element i. In our modeling approaches this subset was usually large, consisting of at least hundreds of neurons, and it was selected at random for each i. The parameters μ_{ij} represent variable *long-range interconnections,* in fact efficacies of those synapses that connect element j with element i. *These efficacies are now assumed variable according to Equation 2,* whereby, however, ξ must be replaced by η_j (which is presynaptic to η_i).

Actually there is no significant loss of generality if function $F(\cdot)$ is assumed linear; nonlinear effects, like threshold, might only cause well-understandable effects in signal transfer like suppressing noise background.

SIMULATIONS

There exists no feature yet in the preceding model that would make it able to store timed sequences of signals. Delayed feedback of signals would easily implement this. However, to restrict the discussion to the basic selective recall operation, we have demonstrated the associative memory function of this network model using strictly *spatial patterns*. To this end we have defined a set of test patterns, stationary two-dimensional images with picture point intensities corresponding to the φ_i variables in Equation 4. It is to be emphasized that *we do not describe the animal visual system in this work;* there are no parts in this model that would correspond to the retina, LGB, etc. Nonetheless we have used photographlike images as signal patterns simply because: (1) the quality of their recollections is easily estimable by visual inspection; and (2) such images contain many statistically interesting details in their internal structures the recollection of which gives us a good insight into the capacity of this model. The images, 500 in number, were digitized photographs of different persons collected by an automatic video input to a computer. The sizes of the picture points are directly proportional to the φ_i of Equation 4. The function $F(\cdot)$ could simply be assumed linear *although even this is not necessary, in view of what will be said later about representing the recollection as referred to inputs.*

In Fig. 11.5a we show a sample of the images; the network model was exposed to all these patterns whereby adaptive changes in the feedback parameters μ_{ij} of the network were caused, the latter corresponding to changes in synaptic efficacies of the simulated long-range lateral connections. The changed network was then exposed to a *key excitation,* shown in Fig. 11.5b; this image contained a part of Fig. 11.5a. Due to interconnections, the network then reconstructed the missing parts at the outputs, as shown in Fig. 11.5c. Because the network operated as a distributed memory where all memory traces from the 500 images were superimposed as state changes of the same elements, some imperfections due to "crosstalk" of the stored images can be seen. The selectivity to key excitation, however, is remarkably good. There was an extra feature in this model, which has been explained in Kohonen, Lehtiö, Rovamo, Hyvärinen, Bry, and Vainio (1977) in more detail. The primary input images were preprocessed by lateral inhibition, which enhanced contours and caused other deformations. The recollection in Fig. 11.5c has actually been operated by an inverse transformation that restores the original appearance of the image as referred to the inputs. It must be realized, however, that in a real organism capable of perception and cognition, such an inverse transformation is unnecessary because the system always receives the signals in the same way; the appearance of the primary images and recollections must therefore be compared when undergoing the same set of transformations.

Figure 11.5c corresponds to a case in which every element of the memory array was interconnected with every other one. In order to obtain a more realistic conception, Fig. 11.5d has additionally been given; this picture represents the quality of recollection from a memory network that had fewer elements, and only a fraction of all possible long-range lateral connections were

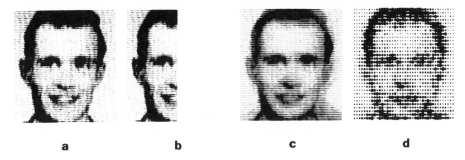

a   b   c   d

FIG. 11.5   Simulation of the suggested associative memory paradigm.

    11.5a: One of the 500 images, to which the memory network was exposed. The network consisted of 5120 elements all of which were connected to each other.

    11.5b: The key excitation.

    11.5c: The recollection obtained as the output activity of the network.

    11.5d: Simulation of a smaller randomly connected network. There were 1280 elements, each of which received 640 randomly chosen feedback connections from the other elements. The network was exposed to the same 500 images, after which the key image of Fig. 11.5b was shown. The recollection is shown here.

employed; these interconnections, 640 to every array element, were generated at random. So Figs. 11.5c and 11.5d, respectively, represent the extreme cases of *completely regular* and *completely random* interconnectivity. Most practical cases fall between them.

It must be pointed out that every picture point or array element in this model corresponds to a column or a comparable group of neurons; the latter may contain, say, 10^4 neurons. The number or interconnections converging to such a group may then be much larger than in this simulation, say, of the order of 10^6 to 10^8.

It may be necessary to clarify that the foregoing simulations were made in the *perturbation approximation,* considering only the first responses to input excitation. To be more specific, lateral long-range feedback, like the short-range excitation, has the effect of continuing retention of excitation and also intensifies the recalled images. Qualitatively the amplifying effect would be similar to that demonstrated with short-range (constant) interactions in the second section of this chapter. Because in the simplest system model it is a linear effect, it is left without further mention here. Another effect of the recurrent activity may be to establish interactions over the whole network although interconnections would not extend beyond certain distance laterally. More complicated models, however, especially those operating in the recursive mode, would require elaborate simulations that were beyond our resources.

DISCUSSION

In this contribution a model of cortical associative memory is presented. It gives a detailed explanation of selective associative recall in a large collection of interacting elements by specifying the critical structural organization required to implement the short-range and long-range connectivity needed for distributed encoding of signal patterns. The short-range inhibitory connectivity leads to the enhancement of contours and increase of the orthogonality of signal patterns, whereas the ability of the network to reconstruct memorized signal patterns derives from the additional contributions of a large number of adaptive excitatory long-range cortico–cortical connections.

The quantitative properties of signal transfer in each functional unit as well as the nature of synaptic plasticity is expressed in a form suitable for a computational study of system behavior.

This model bridges the gap between the cellular and anatomical observations of the neural circuitry and the functional properties of human information-processing system displaying an associative organization of memory. Some of the implications of this paradigm of neural information processing are further discussed in Kohonen, Lehtiö, and Oja (1981).

In the level of specificity of the analysis of neural connectivity this chapter does not go beyond the usual level of contemporary neurophysiology. As the functional properties of neural circuitry are in most cases explained by referring to a small fraction of neuron types revealed by cytological techniques (Shepherd, 1974), it raises an interesting question about the role of this cellular diversity. In the case of cortical lamina at least one hypothesis may be put forward. It is possible that the *form* of the function describing the lateral spread of excitation is "tuned" by various forms of local feedback for which the many polysynaptic short-range circuits involving many types of interneurons may be needed.

As the problem of *optimal selectivity* in signal transformations has been subject to theoretical research for some time (Kohonen & Oja, 1976; Oja, 1977), it may also be necessary to relate the analysis of the present chapter to that. Briefly it may be stated that if one can guarantee a good degree of orthogonality for patterns by preprocessing, for example, enhancement of contours and other distinctive features in images by lateral inhibition, then the selectivity and quality of recollections in the foregoing model is very near to theoretical optimality obtained by the so-called *optimal associative mappings* (Kohonen, 1977). Consequently there is no need to stipulate any more complex physiological transformation mechanisms for a distributed associative memory than that discussed in this work.

For an explanation of the actual capacity of biological memory, in particular the human memory, it seems necessary to incorporate further features like temporal differentiation, attention, and so on in this model (for further discussion see Kohonen et al., 1977).

REFERENCES

Barlow, H. B. Single units and sensation: A neuron doctrine for perceptual psychology? *Perception*, 1972, *1*, 371–394.

Braitenberg, V. Cortical architectonics: General and areal. In M. Brazier & H. Petsche (Eds.), *Architectonics of the cerebral cortex*. New York: Raven Press, 1978.

Creutzfeldt, O. (Ed.). Afferent and intrinsic organization of laminated structures in the brain. *Experimental Brain Research,* 1976, Suppl. 1.

Hebb, D. O. *Organization of behavior*. New York: Wiley, 1949.

Hubel, D. H., & Wiesel, T. N. Sequence regularity and geometry of orientation columns in the monkey striate cortex. *Journal of Comparative Neurology,* 1974, *158,* 267–297.

Kohonen, T. *Associative memory — a system-theoretical approach*. Berlin, Heidelberg, New York: Springer-Verlag, 1977.

Kohonen, T., Lehtiö, P., & Oja, E. Storage and processing of information in distributed associative memory systems. In G. Hinton & J. A. Anderson (Eds.), *Parallel models of associative memory*. Hillsdale, N.J.: Lawrence Erlbaum Associates, 1981.

Kohonen, T., Lehtiö, P., Rovamo, J., Hyvärinen, J., Bry, K., & Vainio, L. A principle of neural associative memory. *Neuroscience,* 1977, *2,* 1065–1076.

Kohonen, T., & Oja, E. Fast adaptive formation of orthogonalizing filters and associative memory in recurrent networks of neuron-like elements. *Biological Cybernetics,* 1976, *21,* 85–95.

Leibovic, K. N. (Ed.). *Information processing in the nervous system*. Berlin, Heidelberg, New York: Springer-Verlag, 1969.

McCulloch, W. S. *Embodiments of mind*. Cambridge, Mass.: MIT Press, 1965.

Mountcastle, V. B. Modality and topographic properties of single neurons of cat's somatic sensory cortex. *Journal of Neurophysiology,* 1957, *20,* 408–434.

Oja, E. *Studies of the convergence properties of adaptive orthogonalizing filters*. Doctor of Technology Thesis, Helsinki University of Technology, 1977.

Rauschecker, J. P., & Singer, W. Changes in the circuitry of the kitten's visual cortex are gated by postsynaptic activity. *Nature,* 1979, *280,* 58–60.

Shepherd, G. M. *The synaptic organization of the brain*. New York: Oxford University Press, 1974.

Szentágothai, J. Specificity versus (quasi-) randomness in cortical connectivity. In M. Brazier & H. Petsche (Eds.), *Architectonics of the cerebral cortex*. New York: Raven Press, 1978.

Towe, A. Notes on the hypothesis of columnar organization in somatosensory cerebral cortex. *Brain Behav. Evol.* 1975, *11,* 16–47.

12

What Do Drug-Induced Visual Hallucinations Tell Us About the Brain?

J. D. Cowan
University of Chicago

To obtain information about the large-scale functional circuitry of the brain is normally very difficult. Microelectrode studies do not provide such information, nor do evoked potentials. Chemical stains, such as 2-deoxyglucose (Hubel & Wiesel, 1978) or cytochrome oxidase (Horton & Hubel, 1981) do give an indication of large-scale structure in the millimeter range, but do not give details of the underlying circuits. Horseradish peroxidase (LaVail, 1975) and similar stains do permit the determination of local and nonlocal connectivity, but the relation of local anatomy to large-scale activity as revealed by 2-deoxyglucose is very difficult to comprehend.

Drug-induced visual hallucinations provide one way to comprehend such relations, if not directly, at least conceptually. Visual hallucinations appear in a great many syndromes: in auras precedng *petit mal* seizures (Horowitz, Adams, & Rutkin, 1967), in *migraine* (Richards, 1971), in insulin hypoglycaemia (Weil, 1938), hypnagogically (Dybowski, 1939), entoptically (Tyler, 1978), photopically (Young, Cole, Gamble, & Rayner, 1975), and following the administering of hallucinogenic drugs (Siegel, 1977). In this chapter only those hallucinations seen in the early stages of drug-induced hallucinosis will be discussed. There are numerous reports of such experiences. As described by Knauer and Maloney (1913):

> Immediately before my eyes are a vast number of rings, apparently made of extremely fine steel wire, all constantly rotating in the direction of the hands of a clock; these circles are concentrically arranged, the innermost being infinitely small, almost point-like, the outermost being about a meter and a half in diameter. The spaces between the wires seem brighter than the wires themselves. Now the wires shine like dim silver in parts. Now a beautiful light violet tint has de-

veloped in them. As I watch, the center seems to recede into the depth of the room, leaving the periphery stationary, till the whole assumes the form of a deep funnel of wire rings. The light, which was irregularly distributed among the circles, has receded with the center into the apex of the funnel. The center is gradually returning, and passing the position when all the rings are in the same vertical plane, continues to advance, till a cone forms with its apex toward me . . . . The wires are now flattening into bands or ribbons, with a suggestion of transverse striation, and colored a gorgeous ultramarine blue, which passes in places into an intense sea green. These bands move rhythmically, in a wavy upward direction, suggesting a slow endless procession of small mosaics, ascending the wall in single files. The whole picture has suddenly receded, the center much more than the sides, and now in a moment, high above me, is a dome of the most beautiful mosaics. . . . The dome has absolutely no discernable pattern. But circles are now developing upon it; the circles are becoming sharp and elongated . . . now they are rhomboids; now oblongs; and now all sorts of curious angles are forming; and mathematical figures are chasing each other wildly across the roof [p. 14–15].

Kluver (Kluver, 1967) made extensive studies of such hallucinations and concluded that, regardless of the cause, almost all simple hallucinations comprise one or more of only four basic patterns or *form constants:* (1) *grating, lattice, fretwork, filigree, honeycomb,* or *chessboard design;* (2) *tunnel, funnel, alley, cone, or vessel;* (3) *spiral;* and (4) *cobweb,* a pattern closely related to those of Class 1. (Fig. 12.1). In addition Kluver noted that the hallucinations are usually extremely *bright,* almost blindingly so, and the *colors* seen are usually saturated. In general the hallucinations do not move with the eyes and so differ from afterimages. This suggests that the hallucinations are a centrally located phenomenon, rather than a peripheral one. This conclusion is supported by other observations. For example, although the form constants can be produced entoptically, in which case they do move with the eyes, they can be induced only by *binocular* stimulation of the eyeballs; thus primary visual cortex (Area 17 in primates and humans) is the first possible site for their generation. Moreover hallucinogens induce form constants even in total darkness, and even in blind subjects (Krill & Alpert, 1963).

FORM CONSTANTS AT THE CORTICAL LEVEL

It follows immediately that if visual hallucinations are generated in the visual cortex, then one must seek to determine their form at the cortical level. To do this it is necessary to compute how the visual field maps onto the visual cortex. Fortunately a great deal is now known about this map. Numerous observations, anatomical (Daniel & Whiteridge, 1961), physiological (Hubel & Wiesel, 1974), and psychophysical (Fischer, 1977), have established that in

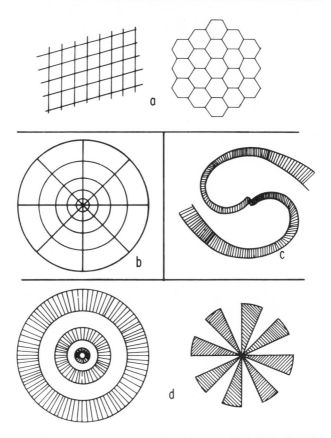

FIG. 12.1 Simple hallucinations. a. Fretwork and honeycomb. b. Cobweb. c. Spiral. d. Tunnels and funnel.

primates and humans there exists a *conformal* projection of the visual field onto the visual cortex. Thus arcs in the visual field map into arcs in the visual cortex. However there is a distortion of the cortical image of a visual object. Small objects in the center of the visual field have a much bigger representation in the cortex than do similar objects in the peripheral visual field. The basic reason for this is that the packing density of retinal ganglion cells falls off with increasing position in the visual field. Since every retinal ganglion cell has its own private line to the cortex [by way of an intermediate net, the lateral geniculate body, where lines from each eye are interleaved] it follows that there will be a differential represention of the visual field on the visual cortex. Thus an element *dxdy* of the cortical surface at the point (*x,y*) represents an area $\rho r dr d\theta$ of the retinal disc at the point (r, θ), where ρ is the packing density of retinal ganglion cells. If this is take to be of the form $\rho = \frac{4\varkappa}{\pi\epsilon}(w_0^2 + \epsilon r^2)^{-1}$, then $dx = \sqrt{\frac{4\varkappa}{\pi\epsilon}}(w_0^2 + \epsilon r^2)^{-1}$. *dr* and $dy = \sqrt{\frac{4\varkappa}{\pi\epsilon}}r^2$

$(w_0^2 + \epsilon r^2)^{-1}.d\theta$ apart from constant scale factors. It follows that the appropriate (local) coordinates are:

$$x = \sqrt{\tfrac{4\varkappa}{\pi\epsilon}} \cdot ln\,[\tfrac{\sqrt{\epsilon}}{w_0}r + \sqrt{(1 + \tfrac{\epsilon}{w_0^2}\,r^2)}],$$

$$y = \sqrt{\tfrac{4\varkappa}{\pi}} \cdot \tfrac{r}{w_0}\,\theta \cdot \sqrt{(1 + \tfrac{\epsilon}{w_0^2}\,r^2)^{-1}} \qquad (1)$$

These transformations define the retino-cortical map and permit the calculation of the geometry of cortical representations of visual objects.

It will be seen that close to the center of the visual field, r small, these transformations reduce to $x = \sqrt{\tfrac{4\varkappa}{\pi}}\,\tfrac{r}{w_0}$, $y = \sqrt{\tfrac{4\varkappa}{\pi}}\,\tfrac{r\theta}{w_0}$, (i.e, polar coordinates in disguise), whereas sufficiently far away from the center $(r > 1^0)$, $x = \sqrt{\tfrac{4\varkappa}{\pi\epsilon}} \cdot ln[\sqrt{\epsilon}\tfrac{r}{w_0}]$, $y = \sqrt{\tfrac{4\varkappa}{\pi\epsilon}}\,\theta$. This is the complex logarithm (Schwartz, 1977). Thus a point on the retina (or in the visual field) may be represented by the complex variable $z = \sqrt{\epsilon}\tfrac{r}{w_0}\,e^{i\theta}$ and the corresponding point on the visual cortex by $w = \sqrt{\tfrac{4\varkappa}{\pi\epsilon}}\,lnz = \sqrt{\tfrac{4\varkappa}{\pi\epsilon}}\,ln[\sqrt{\epsilon}\tfrac{r}{w_0}] + i\sqrt{\tfrac{4\varkappa}{\pi\epsilon}}\,\theta$, for sufficiently large r. Figure 12.2 shows the overall effect of the transformation. Consider now the effect of the transformation given by Equation 1 on visual objects, for example, dilatations of visual objects, in terms of their cortical image. The infinitesimal generator of the dilatation group is the operator $r\,\tfrac{\partial}{\partial r}$. This opera-

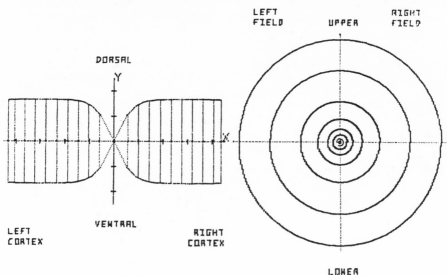

FIG. 12.2   The retinocortical transformation. Right: the visual field. Left: visual cortex.

tor dilates the retinal figure $R(r, \theta)$ when it is applied. Under the transformation (1), this operator becomes the cortical differential operator:

$$\sqrt{\frac{4x}{\pi}} \; [\frac{r}{w_0}(1 + \frac{\epsilon}{w_0^2} r^2)^{-\frac{1}{2}} \frac{\partial}{\partial x} + \frac{r}{w_0} (1 + \frac{\epsilon}{w_0^2} r^2)^{-\frac{5}{2}} w_0^{-2} \theta \frac{\partial}{\partial y}] \qquad (2)$$

The limiting cases are of interest. Close to the center, the operator reduces to $x \frac{\partial}{\partial x} + y \frac{\partial}{\partial y}$, which is just the dilatation operator in rectangular coordinates. Thus, close to the center, the identity group operates. Sufficiently far away from the center however, (2) reduces to $\sqrt{\frac{4x}{\pi\epsilon}} \frac{\partial}{\partial x}$, which is the infinitesimal generator of the group of translations parallel to the y-axis. In similar fashion, the infinitesimal generator of the rotation group, $\frac{\partial}{\partial \theta}$, transforms into $x \frac{\partial}{\partial y}$ close to the center. This operator is just the infinitesimal generator of the rotation group in rectangular coordinates. Sufficiently far away from the center the operator reduces to $\sqrt{\frac{4x}{\pi\epsilon}} \frac{\partial}{\partial y}$, the generator of the group of translations parallel to the x-axis. Thus the effect of the complex logarithm is to transform both dilatations and rotations into translations, parallel, respectively, to the y- and x-axes. It follows immediately that Class 2 visual hallucinations, *tunnels* and *funnels,* when transformed into visual cortical coordinates are essentially *stripe* patterns, parallel, respectively, to the y- and x-axes. It also follows that Class 4 hallucinations, *cobwebs,* map into square lattices parallel to the axes, and that Class 1 hallucinations still retain their lattice properties in cortical coordinates. As to the Class 3 hallucinations, *spirals,* it can be shown that these also map into stripes, the orientation of which is not parallel to either axis. The overall effect of the retinocortical transformation is to map the four form constants into either stripes of varying cortical orientation, or into lattic patterns, as shown in Fig. 12.3.

A FLUID MECHANICAL ANALOGY

This fact immediately suggests an analogy with a well-known dissipative structure occuring in fluid convection (Busse, 1978). When a fluid is heated from below, if the resulting temperature gradient is sufficiently large, thermal convection occurs at a critical Rayleigh number in the form of either lattice patterns of hexagonal or rectangular cells, or, if surface tension is eliminated of stripes or rolls of rising and falling fluid, as shown in Fig. 12.4. The hexagons of course are the famous Bénard convection cells (Koschmieder, 1977), and the instability that produces such patterns is known as the Bénard instability. It follows that a similar instability must be

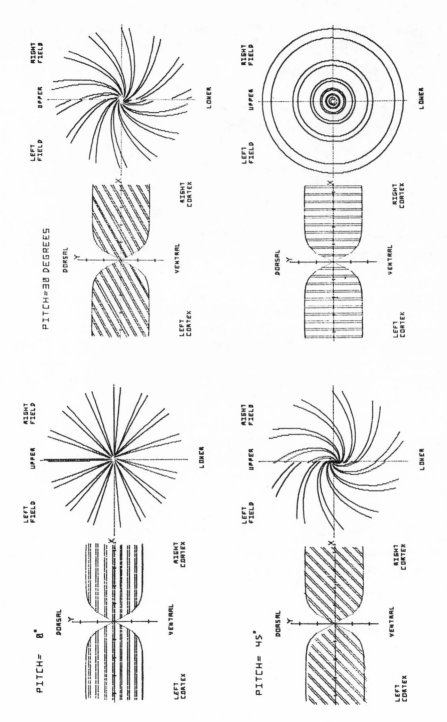

FIG. 12.3   Transformation to cortical coordinates of hallucinations of classes 2 and 3.

228

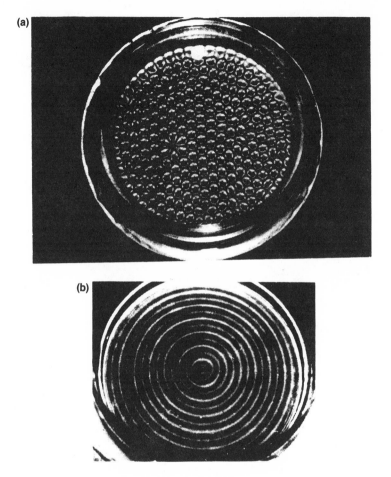

FIG. 12.4   Fluid convection patterns. a. Bénard cells. b. Rolls. (reproduced from E. L. Koschmeider, 1977.)

produced in the visual brain by the action of hallucinogenic drugs, to produce essentially the same patterns.

NEURONAL FIELD THEORY

To demonstrate this, G. B. Ermentrout and I modeled large-scale activity in the visual cortex by focusing not on individual neuronal activity but on the proportion becoming active per unit time in a given volume element of neuronal tissue centered at a point x (Ermentrout & Cowan, 1979). Let $|\psi>$ represent this activity. Then $|\psi>$ satisfies a nonlinear evolution equation in cortical space–time of the form:

$$\frac{\delta}{\delta t}|\psi> \ = \ -\alpha|\psi> \ + \ K(\hat{k})\mu|\sigma[\psi]> \ + \ |P> \qquad (3)$$

In general $|\psi>$ and $|P>$ are N-dimensional abstract vectors, the components of which refer to differing cell types. σ is an N-dimensional nonlinear function, α and μ are diagonal matrices representing decay and coupling constants respectively, and $K(\hat{k})$ is a function of the operator $\hat{k}$, of wave-frequency space. In general σ is any suitable sigmoid function, and the matrix elements of K(k) in position coordinate-space, $<x|K(\hat{k})|x'>$ are of the form:

$$k_{ij}(2\pi\sigma_{ij}^2)^{-1} \exp\left[-|x - x'|^2/2\sigma_{ij}^2\right] \qquad (4)$$

subject to the normalization $\int_{-\infty}^{\infty} k_{ij}(x)dx = 1$. These kernels give the fraction of contacts on a given neuron of type i from all neurons of type j a distance $|x - x'|$ away (Beurle, 1956), (Uttley, 1955). In component form Equation 3 reads:

$$\frac{\partial}{\partial t} x_i(x, t) = -\alpha_i\psi_i + \sum_j k_{ij}(2\pi\sigma_{ij}^2)^{-1} \int_{-\infty}^{\infty} e^{-|x-y|^2/2\sigma_{ij}^2}\mu_j\sigma_j$$

$$[x_j(y)]dy + P_i(x,t) \qquad (5)$$

It is worth keeping in mind a number of points concerning such a representation of large-scale nervous activity. Firstly the coupling matrix elements consist of kernels whose range is infinite. Unless the extent of the cortex is assumed to be infinite as well, even the linearized versions of Equation 3 will not have nice solutions: Long-range effects will propagate in from the boundaries as they do in fluid convection. In reality of course, the cortex *is* finite, and so are the kernel ranges. The finite case has not yet been analyzed however, and I limit the discussion in this chapter to the infinite case. This avoids the problem of which boundary conditions should be used. This brings up a second point. The analysis presented earlier of the retinocortical map is only a local analysis; a more exact analysis would employ cylindrical coordinates to describe the geometry of the visual cortex and spherical coordinates to describe the retina. The local analysis is good enough for the purposes described in this treatment, which is to give the simplest description of the genesis of hallucinations. A third point concerns the assumption implicit in the foregoing discussion, that the cortex can be approximated as a two-dimensional sheet. In reality the cortex is a three-dimensional slab, some 3 mm thick and nearly 84,000 mm² in surface area. It has been estimated that there are nearly 300 differing cell types below each point on the cortical surface (Szentagotha, 1974). However as discovered by Hubel and Wiesel (Hubel & Wiesel, 1963), almost all cells under a given point on the cortical surface signal the same spatial orientation of the local contours of a visual object, and all orientations (from 0° to 180°) are represented locally by about 9 or 10 groups of cells distributed within a block of some 1 mm² cross-sectional area. Visual hallucinations are presumably generated within the visual cortex by the coherent firing of subsets of these cells. Thus the analytical problem involves some 10 degrees of freedom. Even with such simplifications the analysis of Equation 3 remains a formidable task, but the problem is not as bad as these facts seem to imply; the reason is that the emergence of lattice and stripe patterns of coherent activity is controlled by a single eigenvalue of the linearized versions of Equation 3, that one which has maximal real part, and therefore the problem can be reduced by projection operations to one involving at most one or two degrees of freedom (Iooss & Joseph, 1980). The hallucinations actually seem to emerge from the center of the visual field and fill it up in about 2.5 m sec., corresponding to a propagation velocity of 1 or 2 cm•sec^{-1}. If one neglects this and assumes the patterns to emerge as stationary in the field, the maximal eigenvalue is real and simple and the problem reduces to a one degree-of-freedom "bifurcation" problem (Iooss & Joseph, 1980). This problem can be solved by methods that are outside the scope of this chapter. It suffices to note that there exists a critical value of the coupling coefficient μ, labeled μ_0, at which the resting state of the cortex, presumed to be incoherent (Cowan, in preparation), first becomes unstable and generates coherent large-scale patterns. Depending on the circuit parameters, or on the amplitude of any fluctuations of net activity, such patterns are either stripes, rhomboids, or hexagons. In the Mathematical Appendix I give the details of how such patterns emerge from the uniform state.

A CIRCUIT THAT GENERATES STRIPE ACTIVIITY

It is a relatively straightforward matter to devise a circuit that generates a pattern of stripes. One such circuit is shown in Fig. 12.5, and the stripes it generates in Fig. 12.6. It consists of an excitatory population that is locally self-activating, but that can inhibit its lateral neighbors through an inhibitory interneuron and can excite other excitatory cells at longer range. Its effective interaction kernel is shown in Fig. 12.7. In terms of such a kernel, the characteristic wave-frequency k_0 is equal to π/λ, where λ is the range of lateral inhibition, or to $2\pi/\gamma$ where γ is the range of lateral excitation, $\lambda < \gamma$. Such a circuit is closely related to stripe-forming circuits invented recently for other purposes (Swindale, 1982, Meinhardt & Gierer, 1980).

It is possible to estimate the wave frequency k_0 directly from published descriptions of some of the hallucination patterns. Consider for example the funnel form constant shown in Fig. 12.1, and its cortical image in Fig. 12.3. Differing representations of this form constant exist (Siegel, 1977; Oster, 1970; Siegel & West, 1975). In most manifestations they comprise some 15–18 stripes per hemifield. But the cortical image of one visual hemifield extends for some 35 mm (Hartwell & Cowan, in preparation). Thus the wave-

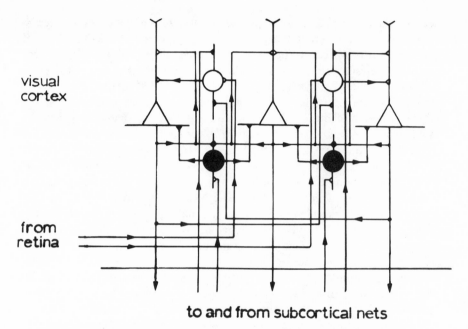

visual
cortex

from
retina

to and from subcortical nets

FIG. 12.5   A stripe generating cortical circuit. Δ pyramidal cell, ○ excitatory interneuron, ● inhibitory interneuron.

frequency k_0 is approximately .5 cycles/mm, corresponding to a wavelength
of 2 mm. This number is of great significance for the human visual cortex. It
is exactly the dimension of human Hubel–Wiesel hypercolumns (Hubel &
Wiesel, 1963). Such hypercolumns must therefore be coupled by excitatory
fibers. It also follows that within such hypercolumns the predominant interaction must be inhibitory, apart from very local self-excitation. This is consistent with hypercolumn physiology (Hubel & Wiesel, 1963). It is also ap-
pealing from the point of view of psychophysics in that each hypercolumn
represents a distinct little patch of the visual field (Hubel, 1977). The circuit
described previously may play a fundamental role in the cooperative analysis
of the properties of visual objects.

PHYSIOLOGY AND PHARMACOLOGY OF CORTICAL
STATES

It is evident that what destabilizes the uniform state is an increase of cortical
excitability. This is what the parameter μ represents. It is an increase of μ that
leads through lateral excitation and inhibition, and the conformal
retinocortical transformation, to the hallucinatory form constants. However, the neuropharmacology of psychotomimetic drug action is not suffi-

ciently understood to permit the exact specification of pathways leading from the actions of such drugs as LSD, marijuana, cocaine, and peyote to neocortical excitability, but such pathways may be presumed to exist.

In this connection, some discussion of current notions of the sleep–wakefulness–attention cycle may be helpful. It is now fairly well known that this cycle comprises three characteristic states: (1) awake and attentive; (2) drowsy and inattentive, drifting into light sleep; and (3) deep sleep, accompanied by rapid eye movements and dreams (McCarley & Hobsen, 1975). I offer the following interpretation of these states. In State 1, I assert that both excitatory and inhibitory interactions are relatively strong. Thus both coefficients $|\mu_E|$ and $|\mu_I|$, representing the magnitudes of the elements of the coupling coefficient matrix μ, are large. Under such conditions it may be presumed that although cooperative activity can occur, the inhibitory interactions will preserve the long-term stability of the uniform state, thus permitting the generation of transient "local" states of activity in the net (i.e., focal attention). In State 2 however, it is presumed that the coefficients $|\mu_E|$ and $|\mu_I|$ both become relatively small, so that no cooperativity exists, nor any local states other than those caused by occasional fluctuations. In State 2 cortical activity is more gaslike than fluidlike. I suggest that in such a state the well-known "α rhythm" of the resting electroencephalograph is a manifestation of such stochastic activity, but this is the subject of another publication. Finally, I propose that State 3 is similar to that of State 1, so far as the cortex is concerned, in that the coefficients $|\mu_E|$ and $|\mu_I|$ are again large. The difference between the awake state and the dream state is not to be found in the cortex, but in such subcortical structures as are involved in the maintenance and control of that integration of brain activities that we call consciousness (Hobson & McCarley, 1977). What produces such changes in the magnitudes of $|\mu_E|$ and $|\mu_I|$? It is known that there exist many small neuronal nets in the brainstem whose secretionss exert a profound influence on the neocortex. Two such nets are the so-called *locus coeruleus,* and the *raphe* nucleus (Hobson, McCarley, & Wyzinski, 1975). The locus coeruleus increases the excitability of the neocortex via noradrenalin (Chu & Bloom, 1974). The raphe nucleus, on the other hand, decreases the excitability via serotonin (Iversen, 1979). These changes are presumed to act directly in terms of $|\mu_E|$ and $|\mu_I|$.

It follows immediately that drug-induced visual hallucinations must be a perturbation of the sleep–wakefulness cycle, in that they occur whenever the ratio $|\mu_E|/|\mu_I|$ exceeds a critical value, termed μ_0. It is known that LSD and other hallucinogens act directly on the brain stem, presumably either to stimulate the locus coeruleus, or to depress the raphe nucleus (Aghajanian, Foot, & Sheard, 1970). In either case the net effect would be to increase the excitability of the neocortex sufficiently to destabilize the uniform state. Figure 12.8 summarizes the theory as formulated here.

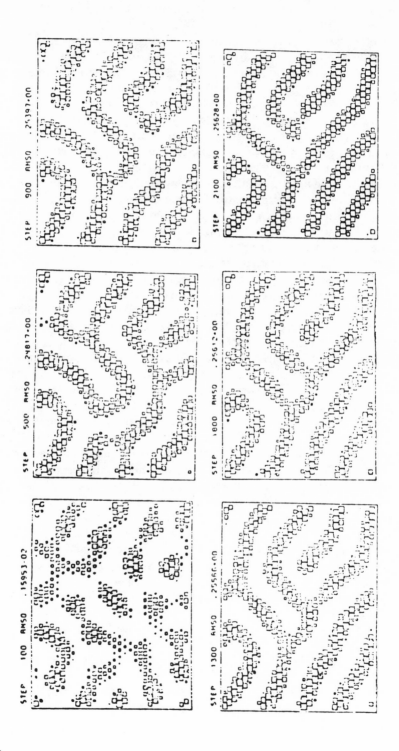

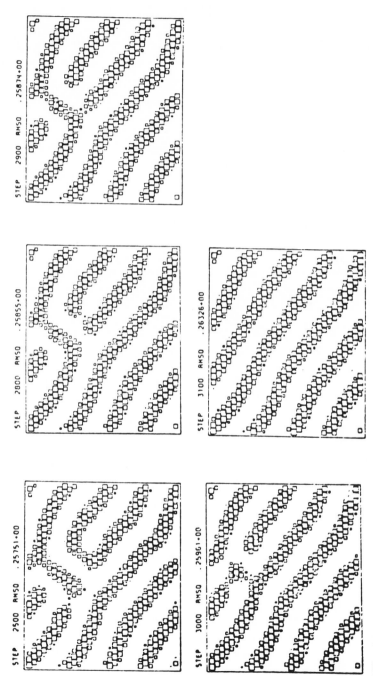

FIG. 12.6 Excitatory activity in such curcuits, showing the formation of stripes from random initial conditions (from Ch. v. d. Malsburg and J. D. Cowan, in preparation.

235

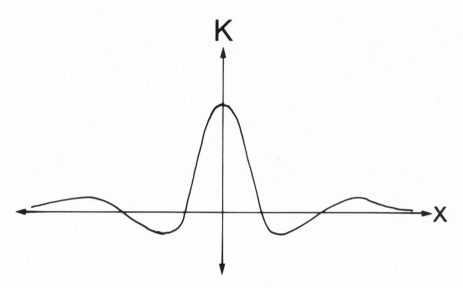

FIG. 12.7   The effective interaction 'kernel' of the circuit.

There is one final point that is of some interest. Electrophoretic studies of the action of noradrenalin on cortical activities have revealed that it seems to increase the modifiability of cortical circuits (Kasamatso, Pettigrew, & Ary, 1979). It may be expected that LSD and similar hallucinogenic drugs will have similar effects. Psychological studies of the effects of LSD on human learning indicate that the drug does indeed potentiate learning. However the retrieval of learned items also requires the drug (Hill, Schwin, Powell, & Goodman, 1977). This suggests that the long-range excitatory connections that bring together the activities of different hypercolumns form part of the substrate for cortical learning, and again that the attention and retrieval systems, presumably based on noradrenalin and serotonin pathways, are affected by hallucinogens. Thus hallucinogens may be expected to perturb, not only the sleep–wakefulness cycle, but also the attention–learning–retrieval process.

CONCLUDING REMARKS

It will be evident that I have skimmed over many important problems. I have said nothing about exactly where in the visual brain hallucinations are made explicit, other than that they must be centrally located, nor have I discussed hallucinations that are not geometric in character. Nevertheless I have given what I believe to be a simple account of the simpler geometric hallucinations, and a possible circuit that generates them. I should emphasize the "generic" character of the theory. Very few assumptions are required to obtain conditions under which two-dimensional neuronal nets will make stripes. Finally I have tried to link the theory to the sleep–wakefulness cycle, and to the attention–learning–retrieval cycle.

MATHEMATICAL APPENDIX

Bifurcation theory, or the theory of the branching of the solutions of nonlinear eigenvalue problems (Sattinger, 1979) has developed rapidly over the past few years. In what follows I summarize the essential features of bifurcation at a simple eigenvalue that are relevant to the problems discussed here (Busse, 1979).

The general solution of the linearized steady-state problem corresponding to Equation 3 can be written in the form:

$$|U_1> = \sum_{n=-N}^{n} c_n |w_n> \tag{A.1}$$

where $|w_n> = |k_n><k_n|U_0>$ so that $<x|w_n> = <x|k_n><k_n|U_0> = w_n(x) = U_0(k_n)e^{ik_n \cdot n \cdot x}$ where $U_o(k_n)$ is the eigenvector corresponding to the zero eigenvalue of the linear operator associated with Equation 3. To ensure that $|u_1>$ is real, the conditions $c_{-n} = c_n c_n^*, k_{-n} = -k_n$ are imposed, and the normalization condition

$$\sum_{n=-N}^{n} c_n c_n^+ = 1 \tag{A.2}$$

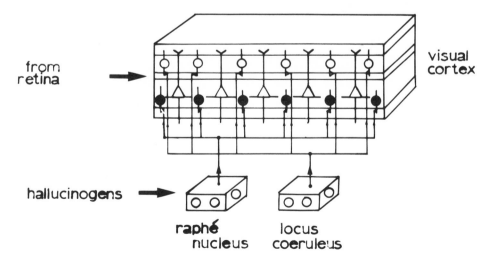

FIG. 12.8   The overall stripe producing cortical system, together with its brain-stem control nuclei, the *Raphé nucleus,* and the *Locus coeruleus.*

The integer N is, at most, the number of differing orientations at each cortical location.

All solutions of the form (A.1) correspond to the zero eigenvalue of the operator $-\alpha + K(k)\mu J$. It is relatively straightforward to set up conditions under which such solutions emerge from an instability of a uniform rest state, at a wave frequency k_0. These conditions require $K(k)$ to be "bandpass," $K(0) = 0$, and that $\det [-\alpha + K(k)\mu J] = 0$ at $\mu = \mu_0$, $|k| = k_0$. One well-known realization of these conditions is the *lateral inhibition* circuit in which each neuron inhibits its lateral neighbors. Of course the solutions are doubly degenerate. There is firstly, the *orientational degeneracy* associated with the fact that neither the initial perturbation, nor $K(k)$ are presumed to have any preferred orientation. Secondly, there is an infinite *pattern degeneracy*, in that the coefficients c_n are arbitrary. Part of the degeneracy can be eliminated by considering the nonlinear problem, and the stability of nonuniform solutions. As a result, in most cases, a single stable nonuniform solution is predicted.

The nonlinear analysis is based on an expansion of $|u>$ and μ in powers of the amplitude ϵ

$$|u = \epsilon|u_1> + \epsilon^2|u_2> + \cdots.$$

$$\mu = \mu_0 + \epsilon\mu_1 + \epsilon^2\mu_2 + \cdots. \tag{A.3}$$

where $\epsilon = <u_1|u>$. On substituting these expressions into the stationary form of Equation 3, a hierarchy of linear inhomogeneous equations is obtained, corresponding to the orders ϵ, ϵ^2, . . ., etc. The Fredholm alternative for linear equations requires that the inhomogeneity is orthogonal to all solutions of the adjoint homogeneous problem. Assuming that the latter are given by

$$<u_n| = w_{-n}, \qquad -N \leq n \leq N \tag{A.4}$$

the solvability conditions yield the system of equations

$$- [\epsilon A_1(\mu_1) + \epsilon^2 A_1(\mu_2)]c_l = \frac{\epsilon}{2!} A_2(\mu^0) \sum_{m=1}^{n} \sum_{n=1}^{n} c_m c_n \delta(k_l - k_m - k_n) +$$

$$\frac{\epsilon^2}{3!} [A_3(\mu_0)c_l|c_l|^2 + \sum_{\substack{n=1 \\ n \neq l}}^{n} [\frac{1}{3!}A_3(\mu_0) - \frac{1}{2!}B_2(\mu_0, k_l - k_n)]c_l|c_n|^2] \tag{A.5}$$

for $-N \leq l \leq N$, where A_1, A_2, A_3, B_2 are structure coefficients, and where it has been assumed that $A_2(\mu_0)$ is of the same order of magnitude as $A_3(\mu_0)$. In the case when k_l and k_n intersect at an angle of $\frac{2\pi}{3}$, the additional condition

$$(c_l c_m c_n - c_l^+ c_m^+ c_n)\delta(k_l + k_m - k_n) = 0 \tag{A.6}$$

is required.

These considerations can even be extended to the time-dependent case (Busse, 1979; Glansdorff & Prigogine, 1971). The key idea is that in the neighborhood of a bifurcation point, the emergence of new states occurs on a slow time scale. Let this time scale be denoted by τ. It can then be shown that the analog of Equation A.3 is:

$$\frac{\partial}{\partial t} C_l(\tau) = \{[A_1(\mu_1) + A_1(\mu_2)] + \frac{1}{2!} A_3(\mu_0)|C_l|^2$$
$$+ \sum_{\substack{n=1 \\ n \neq l}}^{n} A(\theta)|C_n|^2\} \cdot C_l(\tau) \quad + \frac{1}{3!} A_2(\mu_0) \sum_{m=1}^{n} \sum_{n=1}^{n} C_m C_n \delta(k_l - k_m - k_n) \tag{A.7}$$

where $\tau = (\mu - \mu_0)t$, and $A(\theta)$ is a function of the angle θ between the vectors k_l and k_n. This can be rewritten in the gradient form:

$$\frac{\partial}{\partial t} C_l(\tau) = -\frac{\partial}{\partial C_l} + V(C_{-N}, \ldots, C_N) \tag{A.8}$$

where the 'potential function' V is given by:

$$V(C_{-N}, \ldots, C_N) = -\frac{1}{2} \lambda \sum_l |C_l|^2 - \frac{1}{4} \sum_{l,n} A(\theta)|C_n|^2|C_l|^2$$
$$- \frac{1}{3} \sum_{l,m,n} \beta_{lmn} C_l C_m C_n \tag{A.9}$$

where $\lambda = A_1(\mu_1) + A_1(\mu_2)$, and where $\beta_{lmn}/t = A_2(\mu_0)/2!$ for $k_l = k_m + k_n$, and $= 0$, otherwise. As is well known, solutions of Equation A.7 are stable whenever $V(C_{-N}, \ldots, C_N)$ attains a local minimum. The conditions for this are simply:

$$\frac{\partial V}{\partial C_l^+} = 0, \quad \sum_{l,n} \frac{\partial^2 V}{\partial c_l^+ \partial C_n} \delta C_l^+ \delta C_n > 0. \tag{A.10}$$

The first condition evidently corresponds to the bifurcation equations (A.5) with $C_l = \epsilon c_l$, etc. In terms of such an analysis, it can be shown that stripes and hexagons have overlapping ranges of stability and that the magnitude of $A_2(\mu_0)$ is the critical factor of selecting stripes over hexagons.

The variational principle embodied in (A.10) can be given a more physical interpretation by rewriting the potential function $V(C_{-N}, \ldots, C_N)$ in the form:

$$V = -\lambda \frac{\overline{N}}{2g} + \int_o^{\overline{N}} \lambda(N')dN'/2g \tag{A.11}$$

where $\overline{N} = g\epsilon^2 = g\sum_n |C_n|^2$, g a constant; and where

$$\lambda(\overline{N}) = -\epsilon \sum_{l,m,n} \beta_{lmn} c_l c_m c_n - \epsilon^2 \sum_{l,n} A(\theta)|c_e|^2|c_n|^2 \tag{A.12}$$

is a kind of generalized coupling coefficient for all solutions of the form (A.1). The function N is proportional to the square of the amplitude of such solutions, and is therefore a kind of dimensionless *energy* of neuronal activity. In the special case when $\beta_{lmn} = 0$, it is easily seen that V is minimized when N is maximized, so that in this case the realized form of activity, stripes, maximizes the energy of neuronal activity. Of course the stability of the various forms can also be computed directly from (A.5) by evaluating the eigenvalues of its Jacobian. The results are as follows. For $N = 2$: stable stripes, $A_3(\mu_0) < 0$; stable rhomboids, $A_3(\mu_0) < \pm B_2(\mu_0, \theta)$. $N = 3$; stable stripes, $A_3(\mu_0) < 0$; stable hexagons, $6B_2(\mu_0, 120°) < A_3(\mu_0) < 2/5 \ B_2(\mu_0, 120°) < 0$.

REFERENCES

Aghajanian, G. K., Foot, W. F., & Sheard, M. H. J. Pharmacol. Exp. Ther., *171*, 178–187.

Beurle, R. L. Phil. Trans. Roy. Soc. (Lond.) *B, 1956, 240*, 55, 669.

Busse, F. H. Rep. Prog. Phys., 1978, *41*, 1929–1967.

Busse, F. H. In *Pattern Formation by Dynamic Systems and Pattern Recognition.* H. Haken (Ed.), New York: Springer, 1979.

Chu, N. S., & Bloom, F. E. J. Neurobiol., 1974, *5*, 527.

Cohen, A. *An Introduction to the theory of one-parameter groups.* New York: Stechert, 1931.

Cowan, J. D. Neurosci. Res. Bull., *15*, 3, 492–517 (1977).

Daniel, P. M., & Whtteridge, D. J. Physiol. (London.), 1961, *159*, 203–221.

Dybowski, M. Kwart. Psychol., 1939, *11*, 68–94.

Ermentrout, G. B., & Cowan, J. D. Biol. Cyber., 1979, *34*, 137–150.

Fischer, B. Vision Res. *13:* 2113–2120 (1973).

Glansdorff, P., & Prigogine, I. *Thermodynamic theory of structure, stability and fluctuations.* New York: Wiley, 1971.

Harken, H. *Synergetics* Springer, N.Y. (1977).

Hartwell, R., & Cowan, J. D. (in preparation).

Hill, S. Y., Schwin, R., Powell, B., & Goodwin, D. W. *Nature* (Lond.), 1977, *243*, 241–242.

Hobson, J. A., & McCarley, R. W. Amer. J. Psychiatry, 1977, *134*, 12.

Hobson, J. A., McCarley, R. W., & Wyzinski, P. W. *Science, 1975, 189*, 55–58.

Horowitz, M. J., Adams, J. E., & Rutkin, B. B. Psychiatr. Speculator, 1967, *11*, 4.

Horton, J. C., & Hubel, D. H. Nature, 1981, *292*, 762–764.

Hubel, D. H. In *Neuronal Mechanisms in Visual Perception.* Eds., E. Poppel, R. Held and J. E. Dowling Neurosci. Res. Bull. *15*, 3, Pp. 327–332 (1977).

Hubel, D. H., & Wiesel, T. N. J. Physiol. (Lond.), 1963, *165*, 559–568.

Hubel, D. H., & Wiesel, T. N. J. Comp. Neurol., 1974, *158*, 295–306.

Hubel, D. H., Wiesel, T. N., & Stryker, M. P. J. Comp. Neurol., 1978, *177*, 361–380.

Iooss, G., & Joseph, D. D. *Elementary stability and bifurcation theory.* New York: Springer, 1980.

Iversen, L. L. *Scientific American, 1979, 241*, 3, 134–149.

Jouvet, M. *Scientific American 216*, 2, 62–72 (1967).

Kasamatso, T., Pettigrew, J. D., & Ary, M. J. Comp. Neur., 1979, *185* (1), 163–181.

Kluver, H. *Mescal and mechanisms of hallucination.* Chicago: Univ. of Chicago Press, 1967.

Knauer, A., & Maloney, J. J. Neur. Ment. Dis., 1913, *40*, 425–436.

Koschmieder, E. L. In *Synergetics:* A workshop Ed. H. Haken. Pp. 70–79. New York: Springer, 1977.

Krill, A. E., Alpert, H. J., & Ostfield, A. M. Arch. Opthalmol., 1963, *69*, 180–185.

La Vail, J. H. In *The use of axonal transport for studies of neuronal connectivity.* Cowan, W. M. & Cuenod, M. (Eds.), Elsevier, Amsterdam pp. 217–248 (1975).

McCarley, R. W., & Hobson, J. A. *Science,* 1975, *189,* 58–60.

Meinhardt, H., & Gierer, A. J. Theor. Biol., 1980, *85,* 429–450.

Oster, G. *Scientific American,* 1970, *222,* 2, 83–87.

Richards, W. Scientific American, 1971, *224,* 88–96.

Schwartz, E. L. Biol. Cybern., 1977, *25,* 181–194.

Siegel, R. K., & West, L. J. *Hallucinations: behavior, experience and theory.* New York: Wiley, 1975.

Siegel, R. K. Scientific American, 1977, *237,* 4, 132–140.

Sattinger, D. H. *Group theoretic methods in bifurcation theory.* Lecture notes in Mathematics, 762. New York: Springer, 1979.

Swindale, N. V. *A model for the formation of orientation columns.* Proc. Roy. Soc. (Lond.) *B.,* 1982, *215,* 211–230.

Szentagothai, J. *The modular structure of the neuropil.* In *Conceptual Models of Neural Organization* Eds. J. Szentagothai and M. A. Arbib Neurosci. Res. Bull, 1974, *12,* 3.

Tyler, C. W. Vision res., 1978, *18,* 1633–1639.

Uttley, A. W. Proc. Roy. Soc. Lond. *B,* 1955, *144,* 229–240.

Weil, A. R., Mschr. Psychiat. Neurol, 1938, *100,* 98–128.

Young, R. S. L., Cole, R. E., Gamble, M., & Rayner, D. M. Vision Res., 1975, *15,* 1289–1290.

13 Wednesday's Discussion

Cooper: Francis Crick has very kindly agreed to make a few comments on the proceedings of the past few days.

Crick: I did indeed agree but I was asked to make *critical* comments. Now I feel like the man who's been given a very good dinner by his host. The steak has been absolutely marvelous, the wine has been perfect, and then he's asked, "Will you make some critical comments at the end?" He says, "Well, I'm not supposed to have that much cholesterol, and I'm sure you know that alcohol is one of the most dangerous social drugs." I'm sorry to say my critical comments are going to be a bit like that. I hope I may be forgiven.

Before I introduce the rather explosive topic on which I would like to see some discussion, I would like to mention some of the topics I *don't* want to discuss at this moment. For example, we could discuss whether simple systems are worthwhile — but in my experience that leads only to platitudes. I will restrain myself from saying what my experience in molecular biology would lead to, because I know that people find that very boring. We could discuss whether some of the things we've been studying are so unnatural that they don't apply to what might be called natural learning, because of heavy deprivation of one sort or another, or because they occur in critical periods, or because they're massive signals. That *is* an important topic, but nonetheless I'm going to move on from that. Certainly another topic worthy of discussion would be what might be called the possible varieties of Hebbian and pseudo-Hebbian and anti-Hebbian combined synapses. And it would be very difficult for me in any discussion not to chide you for not knowing more about neuroanatomy and what I would call "Lund's rules," which I'm rather surprised to find most people don't know. But it is true that they are only in manuscript and haven't yet been published.

The topic I would like to raise, one very central to what we've been doing, is the interaction between theory and experiment. Broadly speaking there are two sorts of people at this meeting. On the one hand, there are those who really do experiments, mainly people doing neurophysiology and one or two people doing neuroanatomy. On the other hand, there are the people who don't do experiments, but who do a lot of modeling or rather highbrow mathematics. And there are just one or two people who might be said to bridge the gap. The real question is whether there has been a useful interaction between these two groups. Of course, everybody is interested in what the other chaps are doing, but the question we have to ask is whether it is *really* useful. I should ask the experimentalists to speak first because the theoreticians are all too apt to say, "These poor experimentalists, they put their electrodes into things, or they're looking at the anatomy; they don't really know what to look for. We theorists are going to work out the theory, and that will tell them what to look for."

Arbib: If you have a *good* theory, you don't need to look anymore, you *know* it's a good theory.

Crick: Let me just give an outline of what I think the current theory is, and then the theorists can tell me where I'm wrong. It seems to me that all the people doing experiments would agree that, in general, the behavior of the nervous system depends on distributive properties. Even Horace Barlow doesn't believe in grandmother cells to the extent that he thinks that distributive properties are totally unimportant. "Distributive properties" means essentially that, if you want to make some change in the output from a given input, you make it as small changes in a large number of places. The other feature of the nets that have been looked at is that they are redundant. That is, changes appear in many more places than would be necessary for just one simple input and one simple output—roughly speaking, n^2 changes rather than n changes. In addition, the information can be stored in an overlapping form so that you get one lot of information on top of another lot. That is an important general principle. What we haven't had much discussion about is whether the system is linear or nonlinear. The neuron does have a threshold and therefore you get at least a very simple nonlinearity built in there, but a neurobiologist doesn't have to be told that because he knows the system is nonlinear. It worries him, in fact, if the system is made linear when he thinks it's nonlinear.

One of the most interesting conclusions is from the work that Leon reported, the fact that you get really very good behavior if you consider a function which began as anti-Hebbian and then ended as Hebbian. This illustrates what I would call general results; because they aren't applied to specific systems, they are weak from the point of view of the experimentalists. The theories are so permissive that the experimentalist doesn't know what to get his teeth into. If I were an experimentalist, I'd get very irritated when people wave their hands and say, "It doesn't matter if it's done this way or that way." That's what I want to know! I want to know which way it's done! Because the theories are general, they can act as a framework within which precise theories can be constructed, but they are not precise theories of a type that an experimentalist would want.

Another tradition of doing things might be called the artificial intelligence tradition. You don't start off looking for general theorems. Instead, you make ad hoc machines, by means of which you hope you can deduce something in the way of general principles.

If I may speak now to the theorists for a moment, I will tell you what you will have to do if you're going to get any attention paid to your theories, as opposed to polite interest. What you have to do is make a prediction which is, first of all, unexpected. This differs from what is normally called a "prediction" in this sort of theoretical work, which is merely describing experiments that have already been done or making very obvious deductions from what has already been done. You have to predict something truly unexpected. Second, it must be something which is experimentally testable. Third, it must be correct. If you make even one prediction like that, theory will become respectable. But until you do this, the theorists will be talking to themselves and the experimentalists will be talking to themselves. We'll all get together to have nice meetings, but there won't be any true marriage.

I would like to ask first people in the audience who are experimentalists what they thought they got out of the meeting which will be useful for them in designing their experiments. And who would like to start? Jack?

Pettigrew: That's putting me on the spot. I have to admit that I didn't find too many cases of what I would call "strong" theories, that is, ones which have these qualities of refutability and predictability. An example of one might be Rall's prediction that there ought to be dendro–dendritic interactions. The experimentalists had a very concrete test to apply, and they found them. I'm still not very impressed by the special attributes of the distributive system. I accept your point about the need for partial overlap. I'd like to quote something that people here may not be aware of—perhaps it was Barlow's dogma paper which said that laser holography became possible only when the resolution of the film was such that, rather than having a hologram, it became feasible to reproduce the same picture a thousand times over, so that, if you smashed your photograph, you could pick up a fragment of it and see the same picture.

Cowan: At a much lower signal-to-noise ratio.

Crick: Yes, you would have a lower signal-to-noise ratio. Let me chip in here and comment about why the theoreticians have to look at the neuroanatomy and the neurophysiology. One of the things we would like to know from the theoreticians when they're talking about groups of cells is just how big a group it is. There's this very vague talk about columns, which I think is often misleading, for a number of reasons. We would like to know the number of cells in such a group, and whether we are talking about groups in the same place or about groups which are, say, one in Area 17 and one in the thalamus, or one in 17 and one in 18, mapping back to each other, and so on. I don't think the theoreticians have said what they're actually talking about in terms of *size* of groups. In one of these alleged columns you've got roughly 10^5 neurons. Even if you take a subfraction of that, you've still got more neurons than you can simulate even when you try to do an exact simulation. So I don't think we want to imply that there are vast nets all over the place, although it's a very interesting question what the numbers are and how far they go. Would another experimentalist like to comment?

Levy: From the last ten minutes of my talk, when I tried to deal with the forms of the equations that have been used, and from a question that Leon answered at lunch yesterday about the specific requirements of his Hebbian rule, I think it's obvious that there has been very clear interaction.

Crick: I think yours was a good case, Chip, actually. It did seem to me there was some interaction there.

Cooper: One of the things I didn't have time to mention in my talk was that, in the theory I had worked out, there was a neuron that would more or less obey the criterion that Wolf Singer had established. In addition, it seemed to be consistent with the kind of thing that Chip Levy was seeing, because he also has an ipsilateral–contralateral hookup. Without going into details, it seems, at least superficially, to be along the right lines. There are theoretical problems to work out because he doesn't do single-cell recordings, and so we'd have to work out what the consequences of many cells would be under this modification. But then, as he's just indicated, there would be quite a few experiments that he could contemplate that would interact very strongly with the theory. Now, whether they would turn out to confirm the theory or not is uncertain. I agree with your general statement. It's very nice if one has a theory that gives correct new predictions. But theory doesn't necessarily have to give the correct answer. Even if theory gives an incorrect answer, you often can go back, modify the assumptions and then get the correct answer—as long as the structure is clear. After all, nobody really should believe that you can pull the full correct set of assumptions out of thin air. But if you have a clear structure, you can eventually arrive at a set of assumptions that gives agreement with experiment.

Crick: Well, let me turn the question the other way about. If you hadn't produced your theory, would it have altered his experiments to date?

Cooper: My feeling is that I could suggest things that Chip might do that would not have been obvious without a theory. Whether he'll think they're fruitful to do or will do them is another question.

Crick: I think that would be a very interesting test. Of course Levy's results superficially seem to be Hebbian on a rather small scale, that of part of a dendrite. I know you think there's a way out of that, Chip. But you're going to have a hard time showing whether it's correct or not.

Levy: Physiologically, yes. Let me return to a question Leon was asking earlier. The very specific question I would like to ask is "Can the fourth quadrant behavior, the anti-Hebbian behavior, be explained as a monosynaptic phenomenon, or do we have to incorporate a loop?" That's a specific question that I'm trying to ask right now.

Crick: If a theory is promising, and the experimentalists are interested, it then is up to the two to get together to try and think of new devices and new techniques. That's where the fruitful interaction begins. You can't expect every theory to be fully tested immediately. In fact, one of the main purposes of theory is to suggest the best new method to develop, if you can do it. Can we have one more comment?

Singer: I think I learned two lessons about possible interactions. The first is that there is nothing like absolute truth in science. It's always a consensus among competent people — what is considered to be true.

Crick: Well . . . You're obviously not a molecular biologist!

Singer: I think it's very important for an experimentalist with an extremely complex problem to receive some kind of answer even if, as is the case at our level of analysis, the problem can't be resolved to the point you expect in molecular biology. There is a certain amount of convergence appearing between the very different approaches made by the theoreticians and the experimentalists, and I think this adds to the plausibility of our understanding. It doesn't add anything to the proof, but it makes it more plausible.

Crick: You're getting some sort of moral encouragement. But suppose you hadn't come to the meeting and hadn't heard all this. Would your experiments be any different?

Singer: The second point will probably be more specific about that. I think we may agree — or at least it seems very plausible from what we have heard — that the final specificity of particular connections that form the ensembles in this distributive system is a matter of learning and not of predetermined genetic expressions. Thus, details of connectivity will not be identical across individuals. This tells us immediately that we shouldn't go ahead and try to fill out all the details of the synaptic connectivity in a particular animal because this would be irrelevant information. We have to get at more global principles. I think meetings of the present type tell us what we should *not* do in neurophysiology.

Crick: Well, actually, I disagree with you as far as your anatomy is concerned. Of course I agree with your general point; it is useless to look only at a particular small area and look at all the connections in detail, since that will be different on different occasions. But there are certainly very general rules in neuroanatomy concerning, for example what inhibitory cells look like and where they are and what sort of contacts are made where, and things of that type. The point I really want to make is that, if you're going to bring general theories down to specific things in the nervous system, the nature of the nervous system is such that you have to get down from airy nothings and give things a local habitation and name. I don't agree that you can simply blithely ignore all these matters. The question is which ones *can* you ignore? You don't want to look at all the connections, that's true. But you certainly want to look at classes of connections.

Singer: Oh, certainly. The question is the scale at which we have to look at it.

Crick: That's a very difficult question and one that hasn't been addressed at this meeting.

Singer: Well, we had very little neuroanatomy, but I think the emerging knowledge about the projection pattern to cortical association systems is giving us a fairly good handle, at least qualitatively, on the possible structure of ensembles that can be formed by association pathways. We know that these pathways assure a point-to-surface projection, and we know, roughly, the dimensions and the spatial overlap of these cortico–cortical mappings. One shouldn't call all these patchy projections columns, I entirely agree, but the projection pattern that is invariant from animal to animal is worth investigation.

Crick: It's certainly true they're clustered, and it's therefore very likely that the interaction is stronger within these clusters. But you must also look at the actual details, such as the ocular dominance. You talked about binocularity, which is the interaction between two of these domains. They are not *isolated* functional domains—that is a pure myth which has been put about. And that's what the neuroanatomy tells you; that's what the neurophysiology tells you. What that clumping is about is very unclear; it may be because that's the way in which, say, the pulvinar or the thalamus in general projects back to the cortex. The very experiments you are doing show that you are dealing with cells that connect to two of those distinct aggregates, have inputs from two of them. And not only that: If you go to the lower layers, to the sixth layer where you have very elongated fields (the cells project back to the geniculate) they stretch over five or ten of these columns. They must do this in order to pick up the input, to get that length of receptive field. Hence I say that the neuroanatomy at this meeting has been naive; it hasn't even corresponded to the most elementary facts.

Poggio: If that is so — and I fully agree with you, even though I don't know much neuroanatomy — if that is so, what do you expect us to have learned? Why the questions?

Crick: I'm putting Leon on the spot because he asked me to make critical comments! Let me now take another point of view. For example, one of the things that happened in classical molecular biology was that some problems by good fortune were resolutely put to one side and regarded as essentially insoluable or at least insoluable within 25 years or so. One such problem was that of how proteins fold up. We put that problem to one side and said, "We'll forget about that and we'll look at the bit of the problem that seems more tractable." When you choose a problem, you want, not just a plausible set of solutions, but *the* solution — with all due respects to Popper. When you do that, you eventually realize that you can't always solve the problems you set out to solve. So I ask myself whether this business of looking *within* a cortical area is ever going to pay off in any worthwhile way. The folding problem in molecular biology, I must say, is still unsolved, and no doubt will be for at least another 10 years — it's taken something like 30 or 40 years of work to get where it is, even with high-speed computers. I wonder whether it isn't perhaps more valuable to regard each little area of the cortex as a black box, and to look at the interconnections *between* the areas and see whether they are telling us something. We know there are different areas in the visual system. We know that not everything connects with everything else. Only two or three areas project back to Area 17 in the owl monkey, as far as I know. They are interconnected in a special way. It may be, therefore, that it's better to apply theory at a different level. What the experimentalists want, if I may safely speak for them, is guidance. When they put an electrode into Area M in the owl monkey, they would like to be told what to look for. That would be very useful to them.

Poggio: I object to that. Why do you think that we *want* to be told? [laughter]

Crick: You may not *like* to be told, but the theorists believe that you ought to be told. Let's go over this point. When Hubel and Wiesel first put their electrodes into Area 17, a remarkable result came out very rapidly. We can see from their work and from yours, especially on stereopsis, that some progress has been made since. But it is not true that a lot of progress is being made now; the original work was done in 1958 or something like that. There has not been continuous rapid progress; it's been tailing off. It is fair to say that it would be nice if somebody had new ideas about what you should look for when you put electrodes into things and also new ways of interpreting the neuroanatomy. I am on the side of the theorists from that point of view.

Cooper: I think that, whenever you choose a system to look at and neglect some aspects in favor of others, you take the risk that you've neglected the important thing. And we know we take that risk. Yesterday Murray Sherman asked a question concerning what should happen, according to the theory I presented, to certain cells in the monocular region. I didn't give an answer not because I felt that our theoretical considerations have nothing to say about that, but rather that I first had better find out everything about the anatomy of that system, find out exactly what it looks like. Then we will see what kind of answer theory gives. Perhaps it will give an answer that's relevant to what he sees, and perhaps not. But in either case we'll learn something.

Edelman: Maybe the implication of your remarks is that Francis has been going from theorist to experimentalist, but the direction should be the other way around.

Cooper: It's always most fruitful when it goes back and forth.

Edelman: There's a very famous statement in immunology: In immunology, there are two kinds of immunologists — Cis-immunologists and Trans-immunologists. The Cis work on the molecules, the Trans on the cells, and the Cis always speak to the Trans, but the Trans never speak back.

Kohonen: I would like to point out that nobody has yet found the site of memory; no physiologist or anatomist has indicated where memory is. And yet theorists are predicting that.

Crick: If it could be shown that the major seat of memory — I wouldn't want to say *the* seat of memory — the major seat of memory was the neck of the spine, for example, that would be a real contribution.

Let me make another remark: In general, you do not prove things by one method. Before you actually home in on the right answer, multiple methods have to be used. When you come in for the kill, and you want to prove a theory, it's the biochemist and the molecular biologists who will provide the additional evidence which you'll need to make a really concrete proof.

I'd like to add a word about Lund's rules. There are two types of synapses: Type I and Type II. Type I, which have round vesicles and are asymmetrical, are strongly suspected to be the ones that excite. Type II synapses have flattened vesicles and are symmetrical. It's believed that they inhibit. I'm going to go beyond her rules and imply that the identification with excitation and inhibition is correct, although she is reluctant to make that jump. Now her rules are the following: In the mature cortex (she's speaking mainly about the visual cortex of the monkey, but I'm prepared to believe it's true elsewhere), all cells which have a lot of spines on their dendrites have Type I synapses on their axons, the ones that probably excite. All the cells which have no spines or very few spines make Type II synapses, the ones that probably inhibit. Added later: It now looks as if a few of the cells with smooth dendrites have Type II synapses on their axons. That's the first point. The second point is that you can count the number of cells that appear to inhibit, the smooth dendritic stellate cells. You can count them, and the estimates come out to numbers like 4%, 5%, perhaps up to 10% of the total. In any case, they're in a distinct minority. They're also of distinctly different types. And they are not exactly the types that you'd expect to give the inhibition that you would like, Professor Kohonen. There are chandelier cells, for example, whose axons go in very privileged positions locally. There are a few which spread much sideways. In other words, there are a number of distinct types.

Now, Lund claims that if you look at the smooth stellates (that we think inhibit), their somata always have a mixture of Type I and Type II synapses. She further claims that all the other cells, those with spines, only have Type II synapses on their somata. You appear to have very little if any excitation on the soma itself. These seem to me to be extremely important rules. And they raise the question: If spines are the seat of memory, why are they only on the cells whose axons excite? We should very much like to know if someone can produce a general theory that would "predict" that result — not a carpentered theory, you understand, but one which comes out of some reasonable hypotheses about the nature of the system and how it should work.

Kohonen: If I understood you correctly, you think that I claim the memory to be in the inhibitory synapses. In the model that I just described, it was in the excitatory synapses, in particular, those which have spines.

Crick: That's perfectly true, but the synapses where you are putting the memory are ones at some far distance, and yet the spines are all over the place, not just there. And it isn't true, incidentally, that the *non*specific innervation goes by those rules. It's those collaterals that give the excitation at the wings. The nonspecific innervation is all over the place and is not known to be clumped in any way.

The other thing which ought to be said is that the input to the cortex (I'll take the visual cortex again) is a minute fraction of the total number of synapses. Even if you look at the spiny stellates in Layer 4, which are about 16% of all the cells and which are the major thalamic recipients, only about 10% on the average get a thalamic input from the geniculate. Maybe it could be put up to 20%; some people would claim 30%. In any case, *most* of the input to these particular cells is not coming from outside. It's coming from inside the cortex. The same is true in the somatosensory cortex, where it's actually been counted for one cell, which has been reconstructed.

Kohonen: It is completely all right if feedback comes intracortically (even to basal dendrites) because there is no requirement in the model that it come through the white matter and to faraway dendrites. About nonspecific afferents I know only what the anatomists and the physiologists are saying, for instance, what Professor Shepherd tells in his book about the distribution of connections that nonspecific afferents make on pyramidal cells[1], or what the anatomist Braitenberg says about the volume of white matter.[2] If we cannot rely on their data how can we ourselves know anything about this?

Crick: As somebody who has worked in these sorts of situations for many years, I should tell you that the first thing you have to learn, if you're doing theory, is you mustn't believe a word that anybody else tells you. When Jim and I were working on DNA and had got the base pairing, we went over to the local expert and asked him about Chargaff's rule that the base ratios are one-to-one. And he said to us, "Whatever those ratios are, they're not one-to-one." You just have to realize that you cannot believe what people tell you. I know Valentino Braitenberg well, but I don't believe everything he tells me, so why should you? I'm afraid there's no substitute for going over the data yourself, talking to lots of different people, and making up your own mind. If you actually believe what experimentalists tell you, you are lost.

Cooper: The most difficult thing about constructing theory is that you have a lot of data and you have many different people doing work under different circumstances. First, there has to be a very careful perception of what the experiments are, what is really going on. And then there has to be a certain amount of risktaking. It's very complex in the beginning.

Arbib: On behalf of all of us naive theorists, I do want to thank you for your most useful advice. I'm sure that we'll do a much better job now. [laughter] As I understand your advice, Francis, it boils down to two main things: First, we should not do any theory that will not immediately inspire an experimentalist to test it, and, second, when the experimentalist has finished that experiment, we shouldn't believe the results. [laughter]

Crick: The test of a good theory is when you can point to which experiments are wrong and make the experimentalists do them again!

Cooper: To state it a little more fairly, I think theory should have a well-defined relation to what is going on in the world.

---

[1] G. M. Shepherd, *The synaptic organization of the brain.* Oxford University Press, New York, 1974, p. 323.

[2] V. Braitenberg, in *Architectonics of the cerebral cortex.* M. A. B. Brazier & H. Petsche (Eds.), Raven Press, New York, 1978, pp. 443–465.

Arbib: I think you would have seen a totally different picture from the one you have caricatured here if we had concentrated on, for example, retinotectal connections and Jack had brought his model, von der Malsburg had brought his model, and I'd brought my model. I was very struck last week at Neuroscience by the retinotectal session: All the speakers were experimentalists, and yet time and again the impact of models, for example the impact of the Willshaw–von der Malsburg model, was very much evident in the design of their experiments. The next session I went to was the locomotor session. There Peter Getting presented the latest results on locomotory rhythms in tritonia, presenting not only his experiments, but also the simulation results using Perkel's neural-net simulation experiments. When Paul Stein gave his talk, he mentioned the work of Avis Cohen on the spinal cord in lampreys as being one of the most exciting developments in getting a handle on locomotory rhythm generators in the vertebrate. When I talked to Avis afterwards, she said that she had reached the stage where she had actually written and — what is even more impressive — succeeded in getting funded a position on her grant for an applied mathematician, so the study of populations of nonlinear oscillators could be tied into her work. I am currently engaged in a collaboration with several experimentalists working on visual–motor coordination in the frog. We are designing experiments together, coming up with ideas for modeling together — a fruitful interchange.

I agree with you to the extent that I think we have to build interaction between theorists and experimentalists. I think it's important to remember that the experimentalists have lots of ideas. Unfortunately, when the theorist comes up with a lovely experiment, the experimentalist is often a busy man or woman who already has experiments to do. But it is very exciting to see a group of theorists and experimentalists talk to each other so often that they really are concerned, so concerned that there's some chance the experiments will get done. It's very much a social phenomenon, I think.

Edelman: I just want to make some remarks in criticism of a linear theory of scientific sociology. I am basically an experimentalist, and I would like to tell you one brief anecdote from a field whose confines have been, though not completely, still pretty much correctly, established. That's immunology. I'd like to tell you about meeting a certain Australian, MacFarlane Burnet, who I think can fairly be said to be the first man who saw, at least fuzzily, all of the boundaries of immunology as we know it today in vertebrate animals. He came to see me and he told me his theory of clonal selection, waving his hands as theorists do, all very vague. I asked, "How many antibodies do you think there are?" And he said, "Doesn't matter." I said, "Well, what do you think the structure of the antibody is?" And he said, "That's chemistry. If you look into chemistry, you just make things worse because chemistry's much more complicated." Finally he said, "The main thing you've got to understand is that you have one antibody of each kind on each cell." While his theory was constructed primarily to explain everything retroactively, he did make that one prediction. Here I will reinforce what Francis said: His prediction was that one cell makes one antibody, and he made the statement, "If that's wrong, I'm wrong." Well, we went to work and it looked as if one cell *did* make one antibody. But it turns out, as things go, one cell *doesn't* always make one antibody.

Crick: Near enough.

Edelman: Well, yes, near enough. But the point is that his position, which struck me as somewhat loony at the time, was that he didn't care about the details. Now, as an experimentalist, I have to turn it around. The thing that made his theory sensible was in fact the very thing he eschewed; namely, counting what the number of possible antibodies might be. And I think that, although *he* didn't want to imply that, it was strongly implied by his theory. Someone came around and said, "If his theory is correct, in order to make sense, there must be millions upon millions of them. Let's go look." Hence, perhaps in a softer sense, Francis, I agree with what you said — a good theory just sort of points out where you should look, or how you should compound the evidence. In a harder sense, I think that is what Francis is saying, and while it is perhaps overstated, it does provoke.

Crick: It was meant to be provocative. Having got the experimentalists to say a few things, I would like to have one or two of the theorists say how they see where they're going next, especially in light of what I said.

Cooper: The difficulty is that you usually can't concoct an experiment just like that and hope that it can be done. It takes a lot of hard work. What we've been trying to do and what I intend to pursue is to enhance the interaction that we've started between the theoretician and the experimentalist so that we can gradually define appropriate experimental situations.

Crick: Do you feel that the stage of getting the sort of general behavior which you've demonstrated so beautifully has gone a very substantial way and that you now want to take that particular result and look at it in a very concrete situation? Rather than going on doing more simulation on different lines, for example, as some people would do?

Cooper: When I first began, I was thinking along very general lines. I came to the conclusion that everything depended on the types of synaptic modifications one had, and it then seemed to me that one should try to find concrete situations in which one could either verify or deny that. I became very interested in such things as visual cortex because it seemed as if that might provide the concrete situation. As a result, the theory has become much more concrete. One doesn't have some general form of Hebbian modification; rather, one now has the very precise form that has proved to be necessary to explain many of the experiments that have already been done. The next step, as I see it, is to become even more concrete.

Crick: Let me press you a little, Leon. Chip's results appear to show that the Hebbian mechanism operates on a small dendritic region, as opposed, for example, to operating on the cell as a whole. We know that has advantages in some ways, because we have to deal with the problem of how the information gets from one part of the cell to another. Is it possible to give any theoretical guidance as to whether his results are likely to be true or whether they are an artifact due to inhibition, as he suggests? Or do you think the answer has to come purely out of experiments?

Cooper: I would think that is just the kind of question we have to be able to answer. Once we have a concrete situation, given the theoretical structure we now have, we should be able to make some kind of a statement. You have to look at each individual case, but it seems to me that this kind of concrete situation is precisely the sort of thing we want to get into. I think it's possible; I think it's the next step.

Crick: Let me make one final remark in that particular context. I do think it will be useful as you go along to define the various mechanisms and to think, not only on physiological methods, but seriously to think of the molecular biology involved. There may be a whole new molecular biology, and it will depend on what you guess is the actual implementation of these Hebbian-type mechanisms. It may be that the payoff, the proof of something, will come more easily from the molecular biology. If you're lucky, it will support the actual experiments, and eventually the two will react together. What is the substance which is in the neck of the spine, for example? If you're interested in the spine neck, you should know what that is. And I say this to the experimentalists: The more methods you can bring to your problem, the more things will converge to the right answer. Unless, of course, you've got the wrong hypothesis!

Levy: The only way to convince the neurophysiologists would be an electron microscopic study.

Crick: Yes, you're absolutely right. But it is a laborious study.

Levy: Oh, I'm interested in doing the neurophysiology, but, the way science is now, the convincing experiment is the reductionistic experiment.

Cooper: Before we say goodbye, I'd like to say that, though little progress has been made, though we still do not know where the seat of memory is, we should recall that Aristotle felt that the seat of intellect was the heart and that the brain was the cooling system. The point is: It's still true!

Author Index

257

Subject Index